I0065697

Gene Expression Profiling in Cancer

Edited by Dimitrios Vlachakis

Published in London, United Kingdom

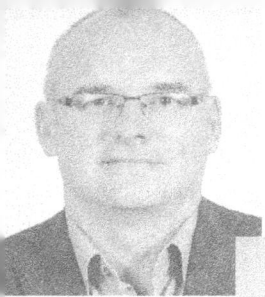
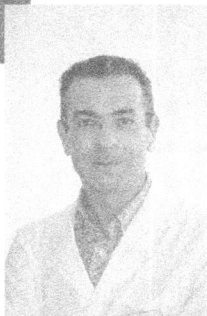
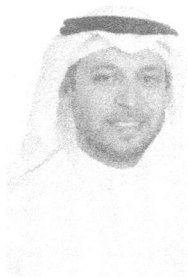
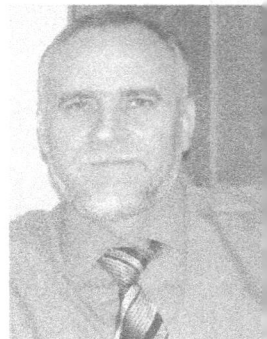
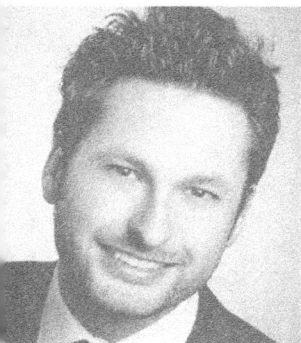
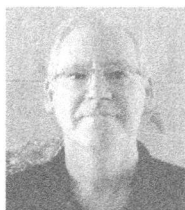
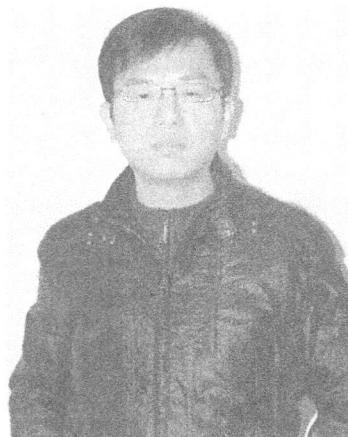

IntechOpen

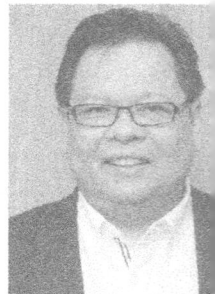
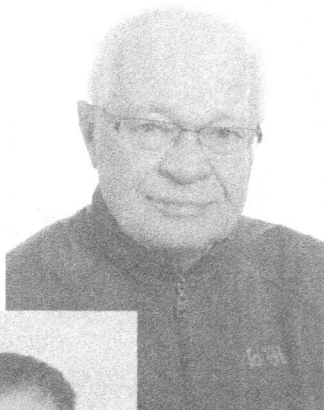
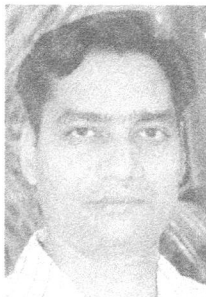
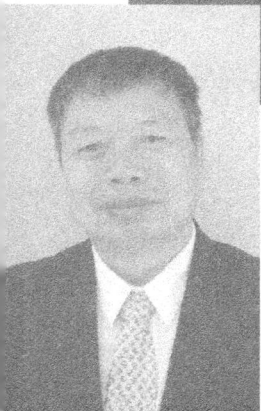
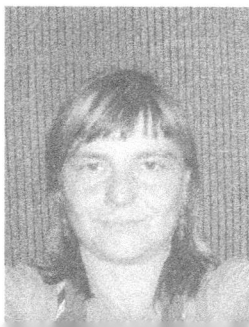
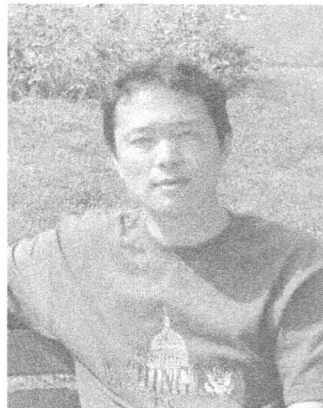

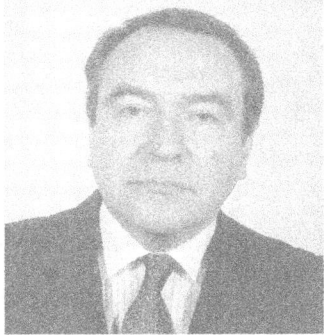

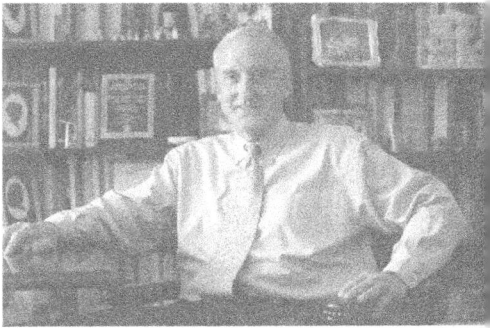

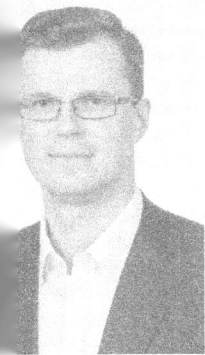

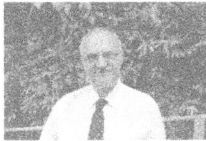

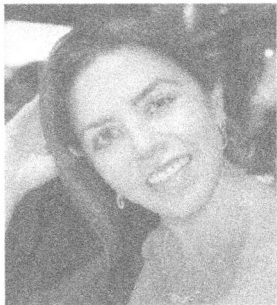

Supporting open minds since 2005

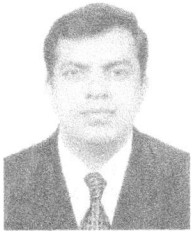

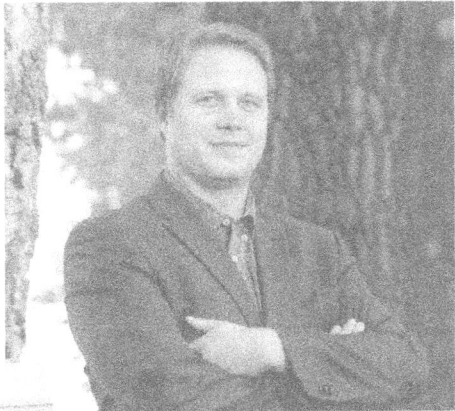

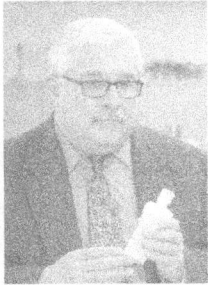

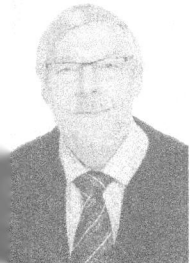

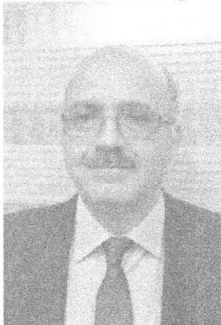

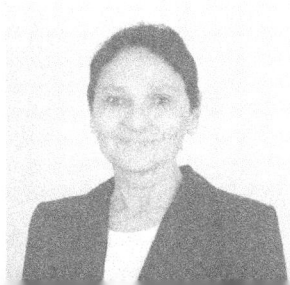

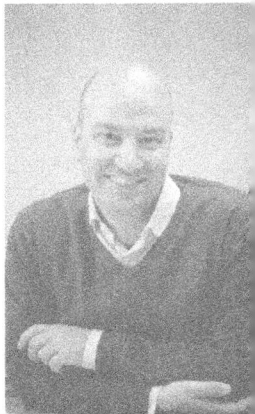

Gene Expression Profiling in Cancer
http://dx.doi.org/10.5772/intechopen.78451
Edited by Dimitrios Vlachakis

Contributors
Zhijin Li, Weiling Zhao, Maode Wang, Xiaobo Zhou, Chanda Siddoo-Atwal, Wan Lam, Florian Guisier, Mateus Camargo Barros-Filho, Leigha Rock, Flavia Constantino, Brenda Minatel, Adam Sage, Erin Marshall, Victor Martinez, Dimitrios Vlachakis, Katerina Pierouli, Thanasis Mitsis, Eleni Papakonstantinou

© The Editor(s) and the Author(s) 2019
The rights of the editor(s) and the author(s) have been asserted in accordance with the Copyright, Designs and Patents Act 1988. All rights to the book as a whole are reserved by INTECHOPEN LIMITED. The book as a whole (compilation) cannot be reproduced, distributed or used for commercial or non-commercial purposes without INTECHOPEN LIMITED's written permission. Enquiries concerning the use of the book should be directed to INTECHOPEN LIMITED rights and permissions department (permissions@intechopen.com).
Violations are liable to prosecution under the governing Copyright Law.

[cc] BY

Individual chapters of this publication are distributed under the terms of the Creative Commons Attribution 3.0 Unported License which permits commercial use, distribution and reproduction of the individual chapters, provided the original author(s) and source publication are appropriately acknowledged. If so indicated, certain images may not be included under the Creative Commons license. In such cases users will need to obtain permission from the license holder to reproduce the material. More details and guidelines concerning content reuse and adaptation can be found at http://www.intechopen.com/copyright-policy.html.

Notice
Statements and opinions expressed in the chapters are these of the individual contributors and not necessarily those of the editors or publisher. No responsibility is accepted for the accuracy of information contained in the published chapters. The publisher assumes no responsibility for any damage or injury to persons or property arising out of the use of any materials, instructions, methods or ideas contained in the book.

First published in London, United Kingdom, 2019 by IntechOpen
IntechOpen is the global imprint of INTECHOPEN LIMITED, registered in England and Wales, registration number: 11086078, The Shard, 25th floor, 32 London Bridge Street London, SE19SG - United Kingdom
Printed in Croatia

British Library Cataloguing-in-Publication Data
A catalogue record for this book is available from the British Library

Additional hard and PDF copies can be obtained from orders@intechopen.com

Gene Expression Profiling in Cancer
Edited by Dimitrios Vlachakis
p. cm.
Print ISBN 978-1-83880-175-5
Online ISBN 978-1-83880-176-2
eBook (PDF) ISBN 978-1-78985-383-4

We are IntechOpen,
the world's leading publisher of
Open Access books
Built by scientists, for scientists

4,200+
Open access books available

116,000+
International authors and editors

125M+
Downloads

Our authors are among the

151
Countries delivered to

Top 1%
most cited scientists

12.2%
Contributors from top 500 universities

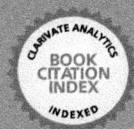

CLARIVATE ANALYTICS
BOOK
CITATION
INDEX
INDEXED

WEB OF SCIENCE™

Selection of our books indexed in the Book Citation Index
in Web of Science™ Core Collection (BKCI)

Interested in publishing with us?
Contact book.department@intechopen.com

Numbers displayed above are based on latest data collected.
For more information visit www.intechopen.com

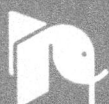

Meet the editor

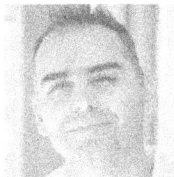

Assist. Professor Dimitrios P. Vlachakis leads the Genetics and Computational Biology group at the Genetics Laboratory of the Biotechnology Department of the Agricultural University of Athens. He is a medical biochemist with postgraduate, doctoral, and postdoctoral degrees in the fields of genetics, medicinal chemistry, and drug discovery. Prof Vlachakis is also an Affiliate Researcher at the Clinical, Experimental Surgery and Translational Research Center of the Biomedical Research Foundation of the Academy of Athens. He is also an adjunct investigator at the Faculty of Natural and Mathematical Sciences at King's College London. His main scientific interests are the designing of antiviral and anticancer agents as well as the genetics and epigenetics of neoplastic and neurodegenerative diseases.

Contents

Preface

The discovery of gene expression profiling in cancer is a relatively new scientific development that has led to a revolution in the fields of cancer genetics, pharmaco-genetics, oncology, and precision medicine. Researchers have been trying for many years to explain the phenomenon of cancer and to discover solutions that will save the lives of thousands of people. Gene expression profiling technology can be a significant tool for reaching these goals.

The chapters of this book provide insights into a repertoire of recent developments, applications, and breakthroughs in the field of gene expression profiling in cancer. All chapters have been carefully selected, adjusted, and fine-tuned in a seamless way that helps them achieve synergy and makes them easier for both the novice and the expert reader to follow. A lot of effort has gone into providing the scientific basis underlying all different gene expression profiling applications, with special focus on the role of noncoding RNAs in cancer. This ensures there is no excuse for misinterpretation of the complex use cases and research protocols described herein. At a time when technology and science are accessible through computers to everyone, the techniques for discovering and analyzing the gene expression profile of cells must be an integral part of anticancer research in the prism of evolutionary biology, genetics, and epigenetics.

I would like to close this Preface with the words of Frank Henry Westheimer: "A couple of months in the laboratory can frequently save a couple of hours in the library." This is especially true in quickly developing fields at the forefront of science, such as cancer genetics, and for elucidating the role of genes in disease. Consequently, chapters in this book have been accordingly curated to simplify the complex concepts of gene expression profiling as well as the role of noncoding RNAs in cancer, without any compromise in scientific quality.

Prof. Dimitrios P. Vlachakis
Agricultural University of Athens,
Athens, Greece

Section 1

Introduction

Introductory Chapter: Gene Profiling in Cancer in the Era of Metagenomics and Precision Medicine

Katerina Pierouli, Thanasis Mitsis, Eleni Papakonstantinou and Dimitrios Vlachakis

1. Introduction

According to the central dogma of molecular biology, the entire process of producing proteins in cells is defined as gene expression, which includes replication of the DNA, DNA transcription into mRNA, and mRNA translation into proteins [1]. Although DNA is the same in all cell types of an organism, each cell expresses only a part of its genes each time, which equates to the ability of the cell to modify the expression of its genome and thus changes its functions [2].

Gene expression profiling is a process in which the genes expressed in a cell can be measured at a specific time [3]. This method simultaneously calculates the levels of thousands of genes leading to the presentation of the expression pattern of the cell's genes [4]. Therefore, through gene expression profiling, we can discover the functions of a cell at a particular time, which constitutes an important application of this method in cancer cells.

A cancer cell is defined as each cell of a tissue in which there is a loss of the standard controlling mechanisms of cell division, resulting in its uncontrolled multiplication, leading to the accumulation of transformed somatic cells, which contain many genetic alterations and epigenetic modifications. These cells have the ability to filter into adjacent tissues, creating metastasis. Metastatic cells impede the physiologic functioning of the vital organs and destroy the physiological tissues resulting in death [5].

2. Cancer cell biology

The process of carcinogenesis begins with the transformation of a physiological cell into a cancer cell as the genes that control the growth and differentiation of the cell are modified [6]. The genes that are involved in this process are (1) oncogenes, which promote cell growth and differentiation, and (2) tumor suppressor genes, which repress cell division. For the generation of a tumor, the accumulation of several mutations is necessary, leading to the oncogene generation and overexpression, likewise repressing the tumor suppressor genes [7].

The genetic modifications causing the tumor development can occur at any stage of the cell cycle. Therefore, an absence of a whole chromosome can occur due to an error in mitosis, or it is possible to arise various mutations in the nucleotide sequence [7, 8].

IntechOpen

The causes of cancer are mostly mutations in the genome of the cell, originating from environmental factors, while about 10% of cancers are due to heredity [9]. The main environmental factors that lead to cancer are tobacco, diet and obesity, infections, radiation, stress, and pollution [10]. Cancer cells can develop and filter through all tissues and vital organs of the body. The most common types of cancers worldwide that affect both sexes are lung cancer, breast cancer, colorectal cancer, and prostate cancer, followed by stomach, liver, and esophagus cancer [11].

3. Gene expression profiling techniques

As mentioned above, gene expression profiling is a useful tool in modern biosciences. The human genome contains genes that can produce mRNA that will later be translated into protein. The human genome also contains nonprotein encoding RNA genes and large areas of noncoding and regulatory sequences [12]. Therefore, measuring mRNAs is crucial in indicating gene expression. Gene expression is essential in determining the cell type, developmental stage, and both pathological and healthy functions. Apart from the ability to present data on the subset of genes that are expressed in different cell types under different conditions, this specific technique can also function as an essential diagnostic test, since it can help record cellular responses to drug treatment [13]. Cancer development, as already stated, is dependent on gain-of-function mutations in proto-oncogene genes that result in dominant oncogenes or overexpression of said oncogenes, along with the loss or under-expression of tumor suppressor genes that lead to uncontrolled cell division. Thus, using gene expression profiling, one can study the difference between normal and cancerous cells to determine the genetic origin of faulty pathways that are a characteristic of cancer and provide potential targets for its treatment [14]. Apart from treatment, this technique can also help with the identification of new biomarkers and gene signatures. Gene expression profiling can be achieved through various assay technologies. Among those, some of the most widespread uses are DNA Microarrays, RNA-seq, and qPCR [14].

The creation of a cDNA library is a vital step in gene expression profiling. An experiment begins with the extraction of total RNA from the biological material of choice, such as a population of cancer cells. This experiment is followed by the use of a specific protocol with the intent of isolating a specific RNA type (e.g., ribo-depletion to remove ribosomal RNAs). The RNA is then converted to cDNA by reverse transcription [15].

Printing cDNA microarrays on glass slides is a commonly used technique. cDNAs are received by amplifying individual clones in a library, and each fragment represents an individual gene of interest. Each fragment is then immobilized on a slide coated with DNA-binding chemicals. These slides can be used in a microarray experiment. In a typical experiment, mRNAs from the two samples to be compared are reverse transcribed and then labeled with two different fluorescent markers [12]. The labeled samples are then competitively hybridized to the microarray. The excessive labeled probes are removed by washing, and the samples are examined using a laser scanner. The relative levels of expression of each sample are reflected by the hybridization intensity which is represented by the amount of fluorescent emission [12].

The development of high-throughput next-generation sequencing (NGS) has revolutionized gene expression profiling. NGS provides the ability of massively parallel short-read DNA sequencing [16]. It is now possible to analyze RA through the sequencing of cDNA—a method termed RNA sequencing (RNA-seq) [15]. The cDNA is sequenced using high-throughput sequencing. The data obtained will be used to generate FASTQ format files which contain reads sequenced by the NGS platform. These reads will be aligned to a reference genome. Finally, the expression level of each gene is estimated by counting the number of reads that align to each full-length transcript [15].

qPCR is a technique used to quantify gene expression and can monitor the process of polymerase-driven DNA amplification (PCR) in real time [17]. PCR uses a thermostable DNA polymerase enzyme to synthesize new strands of DNA. Along with the DNA polymerase and template DNA (in this instance specifically, cDNA), PCR requires primers and nucleotides. The nucleotides will act as building blocks, while the primers will specify the exact DNA product to be amplified [18]. The reaction proceeds to repeated DNA amplification cycles. Each cycle consists of three necessary steps: denaturing, annealing, and extending. The result is the amplification of the DNA sample. Two standard methods are used in qPCR to detect and quantify the product. Those include fluorescent dyes that non-specifically intercalate with double-stranded DNA or sequence-specific DNA probes consisting of fluorescently labeled reports that are complementary to the DNA product and will permit detection only after hybridization [18].

4. Gene expression profiling of most common cancer types

Gene expression profiling has helped in the better understanding of breast cancer biology [19]. Among the applications of gene profiling in breast cancer are the subclassification of breast cancer, disease prognosis, prediction of response to therapy, and specialization of therapy based on the hos. [20]. Breast cancer is composed of multiple subtypes based on intrinsic molecular characteristics. With the use of microarrays, the distinctive molecular portraits of breast cancer have been reported [21]. According to those studies, tumors are classified into five subtypes with distinct clinical outcomes. Those subtypes are luminal A, luminal B, HER2 overexpression, basal, and normal-like tumors [21]. Apart from the subclassification of breast cancer, gene expression analyses have been used to characterize novel prognostic indicators. Some of the gene expression tests for breast cancer prognosis that have been developed are Oncotype DX, MammaPrint, PAM50-based risk of recurrence score, Breast Cancer Index, and EndoPredict [22]. An oncologist should be able to design an individualized therapy identified by maximum benefit and minimum harm through the use of predictive biomarkers. Predictive biomarkers are fewer than prognostic ones. Oncotype DX is a genomic model that can be used to predict therapy response too. Also known as 21-gene recurrence score, Oncotype DX records the expression of 21 genes (16 cancer-related genes and 5 reference genes) and reports them as a single Recurrence Score. The Recurrence Score can later help the oncologist select the best available treatment for the patient [22]. Finally, the next step in breast cancer treatment is using host biology in prediction too, since gene variations in the patient can affect the efficacy and toxicity of the treatment [20].

Lung cancer is molecularly heterogeneous. Just as breast cancer, gene expression profiling has been used on the identification of lung cancer type, while disease prognosis and prediction in response to therapy seem specific to lung cancer subtypes [23]. There are two major histologically distinct types of lung cancer. Those are non-small cell lung cancer (NSCLC) and small-cell lung cancer (SCLC). NSCLCs also have three subcategories: adenocarcinoma, squamous cell carcinoma (SqCC), and large-cell carcinoma [24]. NSCLC and SCLC have different pathophysiology and clinical features, suggesting different molecular mechanisms in carcinogenesis. Genome-wide cDNA microarray has helped researchers to document distinct phenotypic and biological differences in cancer cells. SCLCs are characterized by prevalent bi-allelic inactivation of TP53 and RB1 with SOX2 being a frequently amplified gene and recurrent mutations that encode histone modifiers [25]. Eleven genes have been associated with SqCCs, with the frequency of TP53 mutations being 90%, while 18 genes have been associated with adenocarcinomas, with the frequency of mutations harboring genetic alterations that promote the RTK/RAS/RAF pathway being 75% [25]. Gene expression profile has also been used for disease prognosis and prediction of response to therapy in NSCLCs [23].

Colorectal cancer afflicts about 10% of people worldwide. According to a meta-analysis study, microarray results indicated that the expression of the genes of six chemokines, CCL18, CXCL9–11, IL8, and CCL2, as well as two apoptosis-related genes, UBD and BIRC3, and LAMC2 and MMP7 had an increase in colorectal cancer [26]. Precisely, the expression of CCL18 constitutes an indication of colorectal cancer [27], while the expression of CXCL9–11 increases the ability of cancer cells for migratory [28]. Moreover, the results of a bioinformatical analysis indicate that the influenced genes were associated with chemokines, cell cycle, and G protein-coupled receptor signaling pathways [29]. According to this research, the main genes, which are involved in cell cycle process and transformed in cancer, were the cyclins CCNB1 and CCNA2, the cyclin-dependent kinase 1 (CDK1), CENPE, KIF20A, and MAD2L1 [30]. Respectively, the genes of chemokines, which are influenced by cancer, were CXCL1, CXCL2, CXCL6, CXCL8, and CXCL12 [29].

Another type of cancer with a high frequency is prostate cancer. This cancer is an adenocarcinoma. Its main symptoms are pain, difficulty in passing urine, hematuria, and erectile dysfunction. Its main causes are obesity and diet rich in meat, family history, and HPC1 genes and the androgen receptor (AR) and the vitamin D receptor [31]. According to the literature, there are indications that prostate cancer may be due to regions of SNPs of c-MYC oncogene, which affect the form of chromatin and the expression of the gene. Furthermore, it has been shown that the BRCA2 gene, except for its association with breast cancer, is also related to the increased risk of prostate cancer. Respectively, similar indications are presented with the modification of the expression of BRCA1 [32]. Moreover, prostate cancer has been associated with mutations of genes that are part of the DNA repair mechanism, such as CHEK2, PALB2, BRIP1, and NBS1 that are likewise related to the risk for breast cancer (CHEK2, PALB2, BRIP1) [33–35] and Nijmegen breakage syndrome (NBS1) [36].

5. Conclusions

All in all, many genes are affected and can be employed as biomarkers for the prognosis and the prediction of therapy's outcomes for all types of cancer. Some examples of these genes have been mentioned above for the four most common types of cancer, but they constitute only a part of all the genes that are affected in a cancer cell. By identifying the genes that are biomarkers of a cancer type and the genes that promote tumor's proliferation, the purpose is a more targeted and personalized treatment for any patient that will not only beget the tumor eradication, but it will also occasion the silencing of the genes that lead to tumor creation.

Author details

Katerina Pierouli, Thanasis Mitsis, Eleni Papakonstantinou
and Dimitrios Vlachakis*
Genetics and Computational Biology Group, Laboratory of Genetics, Department
of Biotechnology, Agricultural University of Athens, Athens, Greece

*Address all correspondence to: dvlachakis@bioacademy.gr

IntechOpen

© 2019 The Author(s). Licensee IntechOpen. This chapter is distributed under the terms
of the Creative Commons Attribution License (http://creativecommons.org/licenses/
by/3.0), which permits unrestricted use, distribution, and reproduction in any medium,
provided the original work is properly cited. [cc] BY

References

[1] Crick F. Central dogma of molecular biology. Nature. 1970;**227**:561

[2] Papatheodorou I, Oellrich A, Smedley D. Linking gene expression to phenotypes via pathway information. Journal of Biomedical Semantics. 2015;**6**:17

[3] Metsis A, Andersson U, Bauren G, Ernfors P, Lonnerberg P, Montelius A, et al. Whole-genome expression profiling through fragment display and combinatorial gene identification. Nucleic Acids Research. 2004;**32**(16):e127

[4] Fielden MR, Zacharewski TR. Challenges and limitations of gene expression profiling in mechanistic and predictive toxicology. Toxicological Sciences. 2001;**60**(1):6-10

[5] Kitraki E, Trougkos K. Biology of Cancer. 2nd ed. Nicosia, Cyprus: Broken Hill Publishers Ltd; 2006

[6] Croce CM. Oncogenes and cancer. The New England Journal of Medicine. 2008;**358**(5):502-511

[7] Knudson AG. Two genetic hits (more or less) to cancer. Nature Reviews Cancer. 2001;**1**(2):157-162

[8] Knudson AG. Hereditary cancer: Two hits revisited. Journal of Cancer Research and Clinical Oncology. 1996;**122**(3);135-140. ISSN: 0171-5216

[9] Anand P, Kunnumakkara AB, Sundaram C, Harikumar KB, Tharakan ST, Lai OS, et al. Cancer is a preventable disease that requires major lifestyle changes. Pharmaceutical Research. 2008;**25**(9):2097-2116

[10] Islami F, Goding Sauer A, Miller KD, Siegel RL, Fedewa SA, Jacobs EJ, et al. Proportion and number of cancer cases and deaths attributable to potentially modifiable risk factors in the United States. 2018;**68**(1):31-54

[11] Bray F, Ferlay J, Soerjomataram I, Siegel RL, Torre LA, Jemal A. Global cancer statistics 2018: GLOBOCAN estimates of incidence and mortality worldwide for 36 cancers in 185 countries. CA: A Cancer Journal for Clinicians. 2018;**68**(6):394-424

[12] Sealfon SC, Chu TT. RNA and DNA microarrays. Methods in Molecular Biology (Clifton, NJ). 2011;**671**:3-34

[13] Ben-Dor A, Bruhn L, Friedman N, Nachman I, Schummer M, Yakhini Z. Tissue classification with gene expression profiles. Journal of Computational Biology: A Journal of Computational Molecular Cell Biology. 2000;**7**(3-4):559-583

[14] Narrandes S, Xu W. Gene expression detection assay for cancer clinical use. Journal of Cancer. 2018;**9**(13):2249-2265

[15] Kukurba KR, Montgomery SB. RNA sequencing and analysis. Cold Spring Harbor Protocols. 2015;**2015**(11):951-969

[16] Hurd PJ, Nelson CJ. Advantages of next-generation sequencing versus the microarray in epigenetic research. Briefings in Functional Genomics & Proteomics. 2009;**8**(3):174-183

[17] Kuang J, Yan X, Genders AJ. An overview of technical considerations when using quantitative real-time PCR analysis of gene expression in human exercise research. PLoS One. 2018;**13**(5):e0196438

[18] Garibyan L, Avashia N. Polymerase chain reaction. The Journal of Investigative Dermatology. 2013;**133**(3):1-4

[19] Stadler ZK, Come SE. Review of gene-expression profiling and its clinical use in breast cancer. Critical Reviews in Oncology/Hematology. 2009;**69**(1):1-11

[20] Bao T, Davidson NE. Gene expression profiling of breast cancer. Advances in surgery. 2008;**42**:249-260

[21] Dai X, Li T, Bai Z, Yang Y, Liu X, Zhan J, et al. Breast cancer intrinsic subtype classification, clinical use, and future trends. American Journal of Cancer Research. 2015;**5**(10):2929-2943

[22] Guler EN. Gene expression profiling in breast cancer and its effect on therapy selection in early-stage breast cancer. European Journal of Breast Health. 2017;**13**(4):168-174

[23] Santos ES, Blaya M, Raez LE. Gene expression profiling and non-small-cell lung cancer: Where are we now? Clinical Lung Cancer. 2009;**10**(3):168-173

[24] Taniwaki M, Daigo Y, Ishikawa N, Takano A, Tsunoda T, Yasui W, et al. Gene expression profiles of small-cell lung cancers: Molecular signatures of lung cancer. International Journal of Oncology. 2006;**29**(3):567-575

[25] Inamura K. Lung cancer: Understanding its molecular pathology and the 2015 WHO classification. Frontiers in Oncology. 2017;7:193

[26] Kobayashi T, Masaki T, Nozaki E, Sugiyama M, Nagashima F, Furuse J, et al. Microarray analysis of gene expression at the tumor front of colon cancer. Anticancer Research. 2015;**35**(12):6577-6581

[27] Yuan R, Chen Y, He X, Wu X, Ke J, Zou Y, et al. CCL18 as an independent favorable prognostic biomarker in patients with colorectal cancer. The Journal of Surgical Research. 2013;**183**(1):163-169

[28] Billottet C, Quemener C, Bikfalvi A. CXCR3, a double-edged sword in tumor progression and angiogenesis. Biochimica et Biophysica Acta. 2013;**1836**(2):287-295

[29] Guo Y, Bao Y, Ma M, Yang W. Identification of key candidate genes and pathways in colorectal cancer by integrated bioinformatical analysis. International Journal of Molecular Sciences. 2017;**18**(4):722

[30] Hanahan D, Weinberg RA. Hallmarks of cancer: The next generation. Cell. 2011;**144**(5):646-674

[31] Deng X, Shao G, Zhang HT, Li C, Zhang D, Cheng L, et al. Protein arginine methyltransferase 5 functions as an epigenetic activator of the androgen receptor to promote prostate cancer cell growth. Oncogene. 2017;**36**(9):1223-1231

[32] Attard G, Parker C, Eeles RA, Schroder F, Tomlins SA, Tannock I, et al. Prostate cancer. Lancet (London, England). 2016;**387**(10013):70-82

[33] Cybulski C, Huzarski T, Gorski B, Masojc B, Mierzejewski M, Debniak T, et al. A novel founder CHEK2 mutation is associated with increased prostate cancer risk. Cancer Research. 2004;**64**(8):2677-2679

[34] Erkko H, Xia B, Nikkila J, Schleutker J, Syrjakoski K, Mannermaa A, et al. A recurrent mutation in PALB2 in Finnish cancer families. Nature. 2007;**446**(7133):316-319

[35] Kote-Jarai Z, Jugurnauth S, Mulholland S, Leongamornlert DA, Guy M, Edwards S, et al. A recurrent truncating germline mutation in the BRIP1/FANCJ gene and susceptibility to prostate cancer. British Journal of Cancer. 2009;**100**(2):426-430

[36] Hebbring SJ, Fredriksson H, White KA, Maier C, Ewing C, McDonnell SK, et al. Role of the Nijmegen breakage syndrome 1 gene in familial and sporadic prostate cancer. Cancer Epidemiology Biomarkers & Prevention. 2006;**15**(5):935-938

Section 2

Long and Small Noncoding RNAs

Chapter 2

Small Noncoding RNA Expression in Cancer

Florian Guisier, Mateus Camargo Barros-Filho,

Leigha D. Rock, Flavia B. Constantino, Brenda C. Minatel,

Adam P. Sage, Erin A. Marshall, Victor D. Martinez

and Wan L. Lam

Abstract

Despite an inability to encode proteins, small noncoding RNAs (sncRNAs) have critical functions in the regulation of gene expression. They have demonstrated roles in cancer development and progression and are frequently dysregulated. Here we review the biogenesis and mechanism of action, expression patterns, and detection methods of two types of sncRNAs frequently described in cancer: miRNAs and piRNAs. Both miRNAs and piRNAs have been observed to play both oncogenic and tumor-suppressive roles, with miRNAs acting to directly regulate the mRNA of key cancer-associated genes, while piRNAs play crucial roles in maintaining the integrity of the epigenetic landscape. Elucidating these important functions of sncRNAs in normal and cancer biology relies on numerous *in silico* workflows and tools to profile sncRNA expression. Thus, we also discuss the key detection methods for cancer-relevant sncRNAs, including the discovery of genes that have yet to be described.

Keywords: small noncoding RNAs, miRNAs, piRNAs, transcriptome, gene expression profiling, novel, cancer, neoplasms, computational biology

1. Introduction

The central dogma of molecular biology that has prevailed for many decades, states that genetic information flows from DNA to RNA to protein. Nevertheless, RNAs that do not encode proteins were discovered as early as the 1950s [1, 2]. While protein-coding genes represent less than 2% of the human genome, it has been established that ~90% of the genome can be transcribed [3].

Small noncoding (snc) RNAs refer to ncRNA species that are <200 nucleotides in length and can be further categorized by their shared molecular features and biological mechanisms of action (**Table 1**). SncRNAs have diverse structural and functional roles in the regulation of gene expression, RNA splicing, epigenetic processes and chromatin structure. Due to their broad roles, the deregulation of sncRNAs has been shown to be involved in human diseases, including cancer. MicroRNAs (miRNAs) and PIWI-interacting RNAs (piRNAs) are two of the most studied sncRNA species. Here we describe current knowledge in the biogenesis and mechanisms of action for these sncRNAs and their expression profiling in cancer.

IntechOpen

1.1 Biogenesis

1.1.1 miRNA biogenesis

MiRNAs are transcribed by RNA polymerase II to produce primary miRNA (pri-miRNA) transcripts [4]. Pri-miRNAs are folded hairpin intermediary RNA structures that can harbor multiple mature miRNA sequences and even protein-coding exons [5]. After transcription, pri-miRNAs are then processed and cleaved into mature miRNAs through different pathways (**Figure 1a**). In the "canonical" pathway, pri-miRNAs go through two cleavage events: (i) in the nucleus, the RNAseIII enzyme Drosha cleaves the pri-miRNA hairpin at its base to generate a precursor miRNA (pre-miRNA, ~60 nt) [6] and (ii) the pre-miRNA is translocated to the cytoplasm by Exportin-5, where it is cleaved into two mature (~22 nt) miRNA

Types	Comments	Size (nt)	Ref
MicroRNAs (miRNAs)	Evolutionarily conserved, endogenous, single-stranded sncRNAs, derived from endogenous short hairpin transcripts	18–25	[17]
PIWI interacting RNAs (piRNAs)	Largest group; single-stranded ncRNAs; generated by a Dicer-independent mechanism; a uridine at the 5′ end, 5′ monophosphate, and 2′-O-methyl at the 3′ end	21–36	[18]
Transfer RNAs and ribosomal RNAs	Often referred to as "housekeeping" RNAs; take part of the translation process in ribonucleoproteins		
Small nuclear RNAs (snRNAs)	Found within the splicing speckles and cajal bodies of the nucleus; role in processing pre-messenger RNA, regulation of transcription factors and maintaining telomeres	150	[19]
Small nucleolar RNAs (snoRNAs)	Regulators of rRNA stability and function; some snoRNAs regulate gene expression and silencing processes (i) *C/D box snoRNAs* (60–200 nt): catalyzing the 2′-O-ribose methylation of rRNA residues (ii) *H/ACA box snoRNAs* (120–250 nt): guiding pseudouridylation of rRNA (iii) *Small Cajal body specific RNAs*: functions as a Cajal-body localization signal	60–250	[20]
Small interfering RNAs (siRNAs)	Partially complementary passenger and guide RNA strands; involved in post-transcriptional gene silencing through the RISC-mediated degradation of mRNA targets	19–23	[21]
Transfer RNA Fragments (tRFs)	Generated by specific cleavage of tRNA transcripts; (i) *Stress induced tRFs* (31–40 nt): repress translation and modulate cellular stress-response; interact with AGO proteins to form complexes for RNA interference silencing (ii) *Smaller tRFs* (14–30 nt): biogenesis and function unclear; some interact with PIWI or AGO proteins	14–40	[22]
Y RNAs	Parts of the Ro ribonucleoprotein. Involved in DNA replication, RNA stability, and responses to stress	100	[23]
7SL RNAs	Component of the signal recognition particle (SRP) that mediates co-translational insertion of secretory proteins into the endoplasmic reticulum lumen		[24]
Small NF90 associated RNAs (SNaRs)	Interact with NF90's double-stranded RNA-binding motifs and act as transcriptional regulator	117	[25]
Vault RNAs (vtRNAs)	Associated in large ribonucleoprotein particles (Vaults); essential for intracellular trafficking	100	[26]

Table 1.
Classification of small noncoding RNAs.

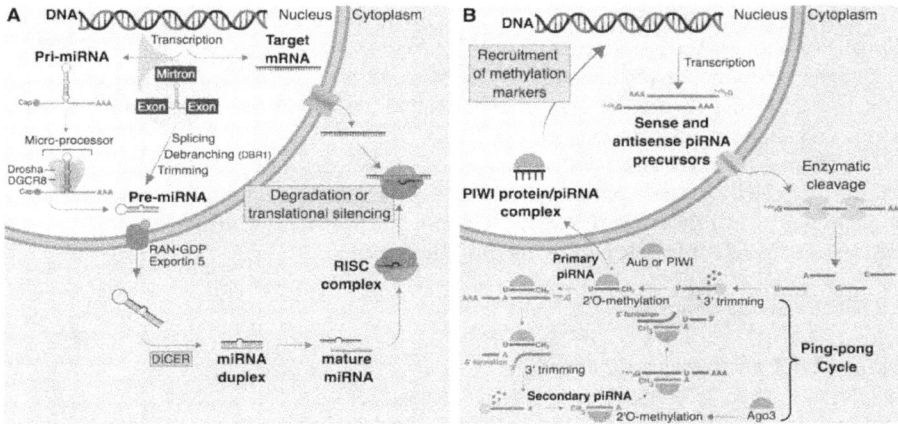

Figure 1.
Biogenesis of (A) miRNAs and (B) piRNAs.

molecules by Dicer (also an RNAse III enzyme) [7]. The major alternative miRNA processing pathway is the Mirtron pathway [8]. Mirtrons are short hairpin introns with splice acceptor and donor sites. In this pathway, a splicing event takes place instead of cleavage by Drosha. Here, the Mirtron and canonical miRNA pathways converge. Thus, the Mirtron pathway is considered as Drosha-independent, but Dicer-dependent. Several other miRNA processing pathways have also been reported [9]. Co-transcribed miRNAs that share similar seed regions are considered as members of a miRNA family [10]. Mechanistically, either of the strands derived from a mature miRNA duplex can be loaded into the Argonaute (AGO) family of proteins (AGO1–4 in humans) in an ATP-dependent manner to form the RNA-induced silencing complex (RISC) [11]. Although one of the strands is usually preferentially incorporated, this varies according to context, and the sequence of the strand incorporated will determine the targets that will be recognized by RISC [12].

1.1.2 piRNA biogenesis

PiRNAs are typically transcribed from genomic regions called piRNA clusters, regions which are typically 50–100 kb long, contain mainly transposable DNA elements and their remnants, and are found in large pericentromeric or subtelomeric domains [13]. PiRNAs are generated by RNaseIII-independent pathways that do not involve double-stranded RNA precursors, through two main biogenesis pathways (**Figure 1b**). (i) *Primary processing pathway*: cleavage of long piRNA precursors, by PIWI proteins, preferentially at uridine residues [14]. The 3′ ends of piRNAs harbor extra nucleotides, which are trimmed upon association with PIWI proteins [15]. Here, the lengths of mature primary piRNAs are determined and depend on the molecular size of PIWI proteins [16].

Upon maturation, the 3′ ends of piRNAs are 2′-O-methylated by Hen1/Pimet, which is associated with PIWI proteins [27]. This modification maintains the stability of piRNAs *in vivo* and can be used as a distinguishing feature in piRNA studies [28]. (ii) *Ping-Pong cycle*: this pathway is initiated in the cytoplasm to produce "secondary" piRNAs. The PIWI protein-piRNA complex (loaded with primary piRNAs) together with AGO3 are responsible for cleaving both sense and antisense transposon transcripts. Secondary piRNAs result from these transposon fragments and are complementary to the first 10 nt of the loaded primary piRNA [29]. This complex shows a strong bias for uracil at the 5′ end (1-U), and, accordingly,

Ago3-piRNAs tend to have adenosine at the 10th nucleotide from the 5' end (10-A). Thus, 1-U and 10-A are signature to piRNAs made via the Ping-Pong cycle [30]. The cleavage of transposons by the AGO3-piRISCs and Aub-piRISCs, and the generation of secondary piRNAs are the main mechanisms involved in the control of transcript levels and silencing of transposons [13, 31].

Each step of miRNA and piRNA biogenesis is subject to regulation [32]. Thus, examining the biogenesis pathways of these sncRNAs through high throughput sequencing techniques may uncover mechanisms of aberrant miRNA/piRNA expression and deregulation in many human diseases.

1.2 Mechanisms of action

1.2.1 miRNA-mediated mechanisms

Once assembled into RISC, the miRNA 5' seed region (between nucleotides 2–7) interacts with specific region(s) within the 3' untranslated region (3' UTR) of target messenger RNAs (mRNAs) [33]. A single miRNA can interact with multiple target mRNAs. Depending on the miRNA/mRNA complementarity, degradation or repression of the targeted mRNA(s) will be triggered [33]. Pairing with complete complementary target leads to cleavage of the target mRNA and subsequent miRNA and mRNA degradation [34]. However, pairing with imperfect complementarity can lead to AGO2-mediated RNA interference. The interference mechanisms include having: (i) the GW182 component of the RISC to recruit associated proteins that would deadenylate, decap and degrade the target mRNA [35], (ii) Eukaryotic Translation Initiation Factor 4A2 (eIF4A2) as a "roadblock" to inhibit the ribosome-scanning step of initiation [36], and (iii) translational activation through recruitment of AGO2 and FXR1 instead of GW182 [37]. Of note, the miRNA-RISC can shuttle between the cytoplasm and the nucleus through Importin-8 or Exportin-1, highlighting the ability of newly-transcribed miRNAs to act in different cellular compartments [38].

Beyond the regulation of their production, several processes modify miRNA function. MiRNAs have a functional role in transcriptional gene silencing through DNA modification [39], deposition of repressive histone marks [40], promoting a transcriptionally active chromatin state [41], and altering alternative splicing profiles [42]. Alternative splicing, alternative polyadenylation affecting 3' UTRs, and cell type-specific RNA binding proteins that affect target mRNA secondary structures can change the available pool of miRNA binding targets. Moreover, subcellular localization of a given miRNA-RISC modulates its ability to bind target mRNAs [43]. These cell-type and biological state-specific factors contribute to the specificity of miRNA. Lastly, miRNAs can be released into and detected in extracellular fluids, delivered to different cells, and so act as regulators in autocrine, paracrine and/or endocrine processes [44].

1.2.2 piRNA-mediated mechanisms

The most well-known function of piRNAs is the silencing of transposons in germline cells to ensure genome stability during gametogenesis [45]. Similar to the lesser-known function of miRNAs, piRNAs primarily act as guides for PIWI proteins and drive histone modifications promoting heterochromatin assembly and DNA methylation [46].

PIWI-proteins are mainly found in the nucleus and co-localize with Polycomb group protein, playing crucial roles as epigenetic modifiers [47]. Knockout of PIWI proteins decreases histone H3 lysine 9 methylation, a marker of repressed gene expression [48]. The complementary sequence of the piRNAs is responsible for directing these proteins to the specific targets on the genome and recruiting epigenetic factors [49], supposedly participating in epigenetic control [47], cell metabolism [50] and genome stability [51]. Alterations in piRNA expression have significant implications to the biology of stem-cells and cancer [52].

2. MicroRNA expression profiling in cancer

2.1 MicroRNA detection

Various experimental approaches can be used for measuring miRNA expression levels. The most frequently used are quantitative PCR (qPCR), digital color-coded barcoding profiling, miRNA microarrays, and high-throughput RNA sequencing (RNA-seq) methods. Material considerations and experimental aims dictate which approach is optimal [53]. While qPCR is efficient in analyzing few miRNAs, array and sequencing based methods offer parallel analyses of multiple miRNAs. Experiments that aim to discover previously undescribed transcripts require RNA-seq approaches [54].

2.2 MicroRNA expression in cancer

RNA expression has been shown to be dysregulated in all stages of cancer and nearly every cancer type [55–57]. Genome-wide profiling has demonstrated that miRNA expression signatures are associated with tumor type, tumor grade and clinical outcomes; thus, miRNAs are potential candidates for diagnostic and prognostic biomarkers, as well as therapeutic targets [56, 58, 59]. In fact, miRNA expression signatures have been observed to be impacted by smoking status in lung adenocarcinoma patients [59]. Furthermore, the expression patterns of miRNAs may be able to supplement the diagnostic utility of mRNAs, particularly in key tumor features such as subtype identification [58, 60]. There are currently ~2400 human miRNA annotated in miRBase (http://www.mirbase.org/cgi-bin/mirna_summary.pl?org=hsa), and it is believed that they collectively regulate one third of the genome [61]. The development of high-throughput deep sequencing analysis platforms has enabled our ability to detect and characterize miRNAs, as well as to identify the impact of their deregulation [57]. A summary of miRNA databases and the tools available for gene expression profiling is provided in **Table 2**.

2.3 Identification of novel microRNA sequences

The annotated human miRNA transcriptome mainly contains abundant and conserved miRNA sequences. Therefore, cell lineage- and tissue-specific miRNAs, especially the less abundant species, may not necessarily be included in current miR-Base annotations [55]. Re-analyses of high-throughput sequencing data of human tissues, cancers and cell lines have resulted in large scale discoveries of previously unannotated miRNAs that are expressed in a tissue-specific manner [55, 62–64].

A wide range of stand-alone and web-based miRNA discovery bioinformatics tools have been designed to quantify miRNA expression and to predict miRNA candidates and their isoforms from small RNA sequencing data (**Table 2**). These tools align the small RNA sequences to reference genomes and predicts putative novel miRNAs precursors based on the molecular features of these sequences, such as their folding characteristics, the formation of hairpin structures and whether this precursor gives rise to the three products of miRNA processing by DICER: a 5'

Resource	Name	Description	Link
Gene expression databases	ArrayExpress	EMBL-EBI ArrayExpress functional genomics data	https://www.ebi.ac.uk/arrayexpress/
	GEO	NCBI Gene Expression Omnibus	https://www.ncbi.nlm.nih.gov/geo/
	Oncomine	Web applications for translational bioinformatics	https://www.oncomine.org/resource/login.html
	TCGA	NIH The Cancer Genome Atlas	https://portal.gdc.cancer.gov
miRNAs databases	miRBase	miRbase 22: the microRNA database	www.mirbase.org
	miRCancer	microRNA Cancer Association Database	http://mircancer.ecu.edu/
	SonamiR DB	Somatic mutations altering microRNA-ceRNA interactions	http://compbio.uthsc.edu/SomamiR/
	TransmiR	Transcription factor microRNA regulations	http://www.cuilab.cn/transmir
piRNAs databases	piRBase	piRNA annotation and function analyses	http://www.regulatoryrna.org/database/piRNA/
	piRNABank	Web analysis of mammalian and Drosophila piRNAs	http://pirnabank.ibab.ac.in/
	piRNA cluster database	Resource for genomic piRNAs clusters	http://www.smallrnagroup.uni-mainz.de/piRNAclusterDB.html
miRNA discovery tools	deepBase	Annotate and discover small, long and circular ncRNAs	http://rna.sysu.edu.cn/deepBase
	miRDeep	Identification of novel and known miRNAs in NGS data	https://www.mdc-berlin.de/n-rajewsky#t-data,software&resources
	miRMaster	miRNA analysis framework, novel miRNA detection, isoforms and variants search	https://ccb-compute.cs.uni-saarland.de/mirmaster/
	miRNAkey	Software for the analysis of miRNA sequencing data	http://ibis.tau.ac.il/miRNAkey/
	OASIS	Online small-RNA detection and prediction platform	http://oasis.dzne.de
	Tools4miRs	Curation of methods for miRNA analysis	https://tools4mirs.org/
miRNA target prediction tools	miRDB	miRNA target prediction and functional annotations	http://mirdb.org/
	miRTargetLink	Human microRNA-mRNA interaction networks	https://ccb-web.cs.uni-saarland.de/mirtargetlink/
	miRWalk	Online prediction of microRNA binding sites	http://mirwalk.umm.uni-heidelberg.de/
	pathDIP	Pathway enrichment analysis by online data integration	http://ophid.utoronto.mirDIP/
	Targetscan	Predict target sites of conserved miRNAs	http://www.targetscan.org/vert_72/

Table 2.
Resources for ncRNA profiling studies.

and a 3′ mature miRNA sequence (and also star sequence), as well as a hairpin loop (**Figure 2**) [65]. Additionally, other filtering criteria may be incorporated to further enrich for real miRNA candidates, such as GC content, seed sequence composition and similarity to known sequences, as well as expression considerations [65]. Therefore, comparing the features of the novel miRNA candidates to annotated miRNA species present in public repositories, such as miRbase, allows for the estimation of the probability of the miRNA candidate being a real miRNA, as well as the confirmation of their novelty [66].

2.4 Assessment of miRNA expression and biological function from sequencing data

To estimate miRNA expression levels, high-quality sequence reads, which are mapped to individual miRNAs, are quantified and normalized for differences in sequence depth to allow for comparison between samples [67]. A variety of statistical tests can be applied to determine differential expression. For example, tissue-specificity of the miRNAs derived from a given organ site can be assessed by comparing expression patterns across tissue types, by using Principal Component Analysis (PCA) or nonlinear t-Distributed Stochastic Neighbor Embedding (t-SNE) [62, 63]. Additionally, differential expression of miRNA between biological states, such as neoplastic versus nonmalignant tissue samples, can be compared using various standard parametric or nonparametric statistical tests (**Figure 3**) [63, 64].

Once miRNAs-of-interest are identified, their function can be assessed through *in silico* methods of gene-target prediction. Prediction of miRNA:mRNA targets enables the understanding of their involvement in genetic regulatory networks. Since one miRNA can target multiple gene transcripts, it is challenging to comprehensively capture regulatory targets without also yielding false predictions. Therefore, a variety of computational approaches have been developed for the confirmation of miRNA:mRNA target interaction which consider features such as (i) seed match, (ii) conservation, (iii) free energy, and (iv) site accessibility [68].

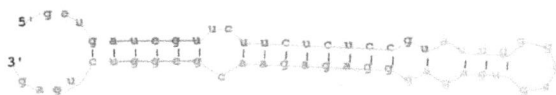

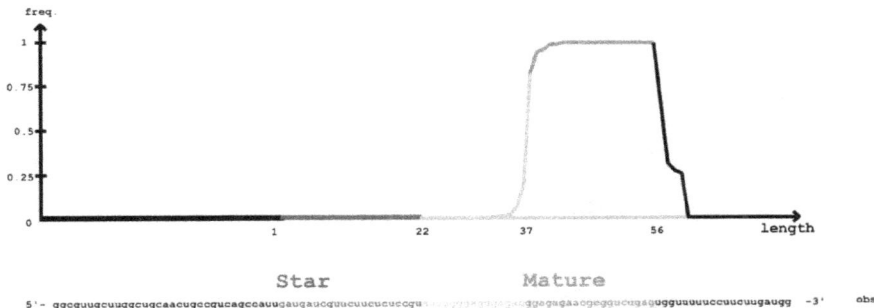

Figure 2.
Output from the miRDeep2 algorithm demonstrates that a previously unannotated small RNA sequence exhibits miRNA-like folding structures.

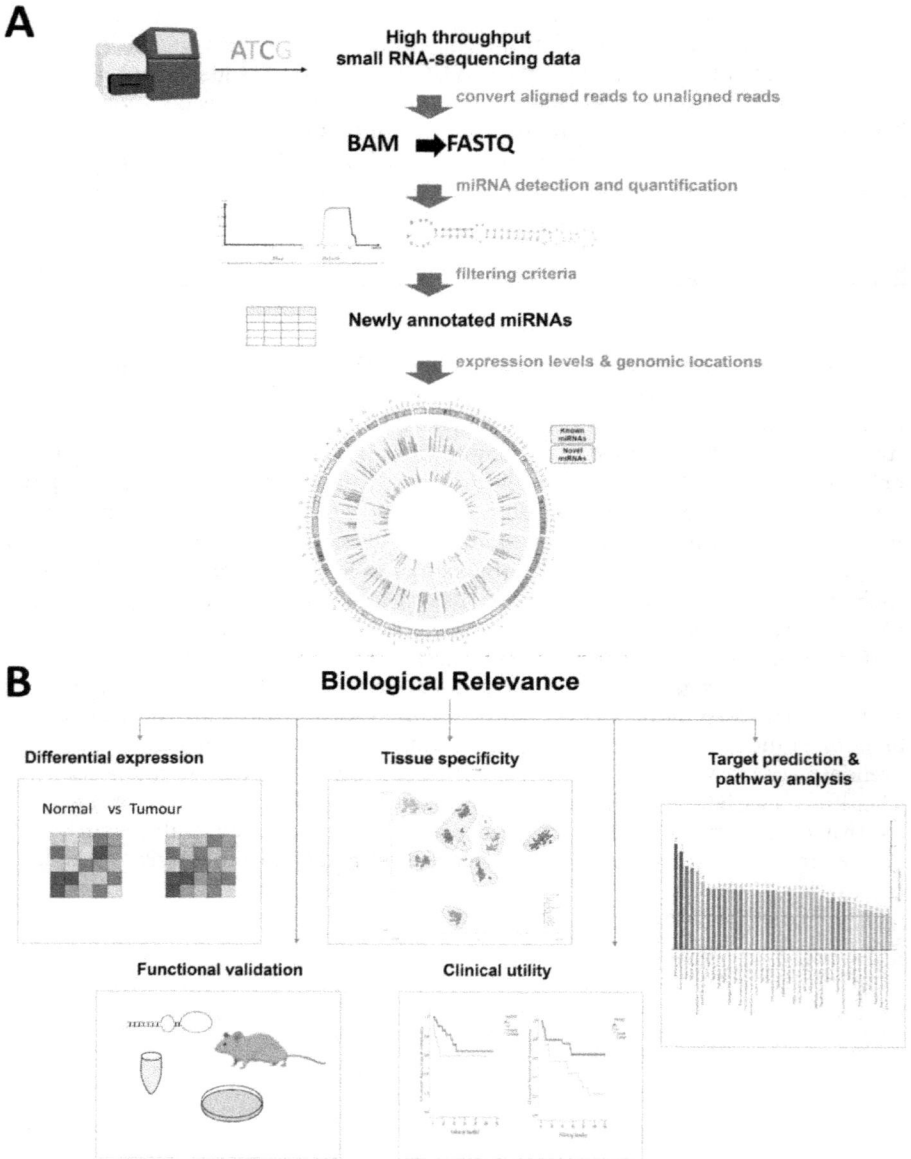

Figure 3.
Pipeline for detection and characterization of known and novel miRNAs. A) An example of bioinformatic pipeline for the detection of miRNAs. B) Main features for assessment of the biological relevance of miRNAs.

The growing availability of high throughput next generation sequencing (NGS) data will not only lead to novel miRNA discovery but will allow us to further elucidate the role of miRNA expression in human biology and disease such as cancer.

3. PIWI-interacting RNA expression profiling in cancer

PiRNAs are known to act in an evolutionarily conserved innate protection mechanism against transposable elements in germ cell genomes [69]. Beyond the

piRNA functions described in germ cells, there is increasing evidence of multifac-
eted action not restricted to transposon silencing in somatic cells [70]. Although the
function of piRNAs in somatic cells and their relationship with tumorigenesis and
cancer progression are still unknown, many studies seek to evaluate PIWI proteins
and piRNA expression in a variety of malignancies [71].

3.1 piRNA detection and resources

Since piRNAs resemble miRNAs in length and structure, the same expression
profiling platforms are applicable, wherein small RNA sequencing, microarrays,
and quantitative PCR are the most widely used. The identification of piRNAs is
mainly performed by small RNA sequencing, through extracting the reads with the
proper length (generally from 24 to 32 nucleotides) that present piRNA-like features
[72]. As previously discussed, piRNAs are frequently identified by a uridine nucleotide in the first position, have an adenosine nucleotide at the 10th position, have
a 2′-O-methylation at the 3′ end, and are mapped in clusters in the genome [72].
Although the expression can be confirmed by *in situ* hybridization and Northern
blotting [73], the co-immunoprecipitation assay is the gold standard technique
[74]. This analysis allows the isolation and characterization of RNAs physically
interacting with PIWI-proteins [74]. However, the lack of highly specific antibodies
for human PIWI-proteins limits the discovery of relevant piRNAs [75]. Functional
studies using knockdown or knockout experiments for newly discovered piRNAs
are fundamental to elucidate the biological role of these sequences [73].

The increasing application of large-scale small RNA sequencing has enabled the
discovery of a large amount of piRNAs. The most widely used piRNA compendiums
are piRBase and piRNABank, which contain millions of annotated human piRNA
sequences—8,438,265 and 11,147,151 annotated piRNAs to date, respectively (**Table 2**)
[76, 77]. Despite the large number of annotated sequences in these databases and many
studies describing piRNA expression in somatic and malignant tissues, this knowledge
must be considered with caution. It has been demonstrated that different piRNA
databases include some RNA fragments that have similar sizes and features to piRNAs,
representing possible contaminants; yet, sncRNAs derived from tRNAs have been
described to interact with PIWIL2 and are deregulated in cancer [78].

PIWI-interacting RNAs regulate the expression of mRNAs by guiding PIWI-
proteins [46]. Bioinformatics approaches have shown that approximately 28.5%
of human mRNA sequences contain at least one retrotransposon sequence in their
3′ UTRs, and those mRNAs can be post-transcriptionally regulated by piRNAs
[79]. In addition, many piRNAs do not match transposon sequences, suggesting an even greater set of targets and functional roles for piRNAs [80]. In fact,
cross-linking immunoprecipitation (CLIP) analyses unveils many nontransposon
mRNAs engaged with PIWI proteins [81]. In *Caenorhabditis elegans*, it was previous
demonstrated that piRNA action is analogous to miRNAs, in that seed sequences
are required for mRNA targeting, but unlike miRNAs, piRNAs do not tolerate many
mismatches out of this region [82]. Potential piRNA targets can be retrieved using
algorithms initially designed for miRNAs, such as miRanda [83], where stringent
alignment ($\geq$170) and free-energy scores ($\leq$−20.0 kcal/mol) are required for
piRNA analyses [84]. However, the identification of piRNA targets is very challenging, as the targeting rules are still unsolved [82].

3.2 piRNA profiles in cancer

PIWI proteins 1–4 and PIWI-related proteins (DDX4, HENMT1, MAEL and
TDRD1) have been reported to be disrupted in tumor cell line and patient samples

[85, 86]. The sncRNA repertoire of cancer cell lines from the NCI-60 panel (59 cell lines from nine different tissues) was recently characterized, where piRNAs comprised the largest proportion of expressed transcripts, followed by miRNAs and snRNAs [62]. In lung cancer cell lines, it was previously described 555 differentially expressed piRNAs and piRNA-like sncRNAs (piRNA-Ls) compared with lung bronchial epithelial cell lines [87]. Among them, piR-L-163 was found to be down-regulated in cancer cell lines and interact with phosphorylated ERM, regulating cell proliferation, migration and invasion.

Interestingly, piRNA expression profiling studies in tumor tissues revealed that piRNAs can be influenced by etiologic factors, such as tobacco consumption and HPV infection in lung and head and neck cancer [88–90]. The piRNA transcrip-tome of 6260 samples (from 11 organs) from The Cancer Genome Atlas (TCGA) consortium was prior screened [56]. Tumor samples presented a higher number of expressed piRNAs (n = 522) compared to somatic non-neoplastic tissues (n = 273), suggesting their potential as biomarkers. RNA sequencing found piR-1245 to be overexpressed and demonstrate oncogenic roles in colorectal cancer, inducing pro-liferation, colony formation, invasion, and apoptosis resistance [91]. Several other piRNAs have been reported to be overexpressed in numerous human malignancies [92–95]. Alternatively, piRNAs have also been described to have anti-tumor effects. For example, piR-39980 was demonstrated through functional assays to decrease proliferation, migration, invasion, colony formation, and to induce apoptosis in fibrosarcoma cell lines upon piRNA-mimic transfection [96].

The role of piRNAs in the response to chemotherapy has also been addressed [97–99]. In PIWL2-knockout embryonic fibroblast mouse models, the commonly overexpressed gene *PIWL2* was demonstrated to facilitate chromatin acetylation and relaxation in response to cisplatin treatment, leading to enhanced DNA repair and highlighting its potential role in treatment resistance [97]. piR-FTH1 was reported to drive chemoresistance in breast tumor cell lines, where its repression could sensitize tumor cells to doxorubicin [98]. Similarly, inhibition of piR-L-138 can increase apoptosis in cisplatin-treated lung cancer cell lines and patient-derived xenografts [99].

4. Emerging roles of sncRNA as cancer biomarkers

Considering the tissue-specificity of miRNAs and piRNAs in cancerous and healthy samples [55, 56], several individual or sncRNA-sets have been proposed as diagnostic or prognostic markers [56]. A set of 24 miRNAs evaluated by qPCR has been shown to correctly discriminate malignant from benign thyroid nodules with high sensitivity and specificity, potentially avoiding unnecessary diagnostic thyroidectomies [100]. In gastric adenocarcinoma, a three-piRNA recurrence risk signature was reported, using the small RNA sequencing data from the TCGA data-base [101]. Similarly, a higher expression of piR-1245 was linked to a lower overall survival in three independent cohorts of colorectal cancer patients [91].

The use of sncRNAs as liquid biopsy cancer-markers is also under intense investigation [102, 103]. In fact, both miRNAs and piRNAs are detectable in human serum, as demonstrated by a recent study based on RNA sequencing analysis in 477 serum samples [104]. Moreover, sncRNAs are enriched in extracellular vesicles (miRNAs ~40%, piRNAs ~40%) [105], allowing for their export from the cell in which they were synthesized to affect cells at a distance [106]. Models based on miRNA and piRNA combinations were able to correctly classify colon and prostate cancer patients from healthy individuals [106]. A four-miRNA expression signature in the serum of triple negative breast cancer patients was also demonstrated to be an optimal survival predictor [107]. Recently, a qPCR assay comprising two targets (piR-5937 and piR-28876) and one reference piRNA (piR-28131) was suggested to detect early colon cancer [108]. Despite the low piRNA levels in the serum of cancer patients, they presented better detection sensitivity than the currently used biomarkers such as CA19-9 and carcinoembryonic antigen (CEA).

Many studies are currently investigating the ability of miRNA/piRNA signatures to empower cancer screening through the prediction of cancer recurrence or progression, stratification of patients by prognosis, and prediction of tumor response to various treatments. However, more efforts are still needed to screen miRNA/piRNA biomarker candidates and further validate them in large cohorts.

5. Conclusions

Here, we summarized the roles of small noncoding RNAs in normal and disease molecular biology and highlighted the importance of developing high-throughput sncRNA-detection methods in genome analyses. Transcribed through a variety of mechanisms, these molecules act in the widespread and specific regulation of gene expression. However, before these results can be translated to the clinic many factors must still be considered, including the development of effective and specific delivery system for sncRNA-based therapeutics and the broad validation of these sequences in large external cohorts. As our ability to detect and validate these sequences develops, we will continue to uncover their biological functions and potential uses in the clinical management of many diseases, including cancer.

Acknowledgements

This work was supported by grants from the Canadian Institutes for Health Research (CIHR FDN-143345), and scholarships from CIHR, Vanier Canada, the BC Cancer Foundation, the Ligue nationale contre le cancer, the Fonds de Recherche en Santé Respiratoire (appel d'offres 2018 emis en commun avec la Fondation du Souffle), the Fondation Charles Nicolle, and the São Paulo Research Foundation (FAPESP 2015/17707-5 and 2018/06138-8). E.A.M. is a Vanier Canada Graduate Scholar.

Conflict of interest

The authors have no conflicts to declare.

Author details

Florian Guisier[1,2*†], Mateus Camargo Barros-Filho[1,3†], Leigha D. Rock[1,4,5†], Flavia B. Constantino[1,6], Brenda C. Minatel[1], Adam P. Sage[1], Erin A. Marshall[1], Victor D. Martinez[1] and Wan L. Lam[1]

1 Department of Integrative Oncology, British Columbia Cancer Research Centre, Vancouver, BC, Canada

2 Pneumology Department, Rouen University Hospital, Rouen, France

3 International Research Center, A.C. Camargo Cancer Center, Sao Paulo, SP, Brazil

4 Department of Cancer Control Research, British Columbia Cancer Research Centre, Vancouver, BC, Canada

5 Department of Oral and Biological Medical Sciences, Faculty of Dentistry, University of British Columbia, Vancouver, BC, Canada

6 Institute of Biosciences, São Paulo State University, Botucatu, SP, Brazil

*Address all correspondence to: fguisier@bccrc.ca

† These authors contributed equally to this work.

IntechOpen

© 2019 The Author(s). Licensee IntechOpen. This chapter is distributed under the terms of the Creative Commons Attribution License (http://creativecommons.org/licenses/by/3.0), which permits unrestricted use, distribution, and reproduction in any medium, provided the original work is properly cited. (cc) BY

References

[1] Stark BC, Kole R, Bowman EJ, Altman S. Ribonuclease P: An enzyme with an essential RNA component. Proceedings of the National Academy of Sciences of the United States of America. 1978;**75**(8):3717-3721

[2] Yang VW, Lerner MR, Steitz JA, Flint SJ. A small nuclear ribonucleoprotein is required for splicing of adenoviral early RNA sequences. Proceedings of the National Academy of Sciences of the United States of America. 1981;**78**(3):1371-1375

[3] Carninci P, Kasukawa T, Katayama S, Gough J, Frith MC, Maeda N, et al. The transcriptional landscape of the mammalian genome. Science. 2005;**309**(5740):1559-1563

[4] Macfarlane LA, Murphy PR. MicroRNA: Biogenesis, function and role in cancer. Current Genomics. 2010;**11**(7):537-561

[5] Cech TR, Steitz JA. The noncoding RNA revolution-trashing old rules to forge new ones. Cell. 2014;**157**(1):77-94

[6] Lee Y, Ahn C, Han J, Choi H, Kim J, Yim J, et al. The nuclear RNase III Drosha initiates microRNA processing. Nature. 2003;**425**(6956):415-419

[7] Hammond SM, Bernstein E, Beach D, Hannon GJ. An RNA-directed nuclease mediates post-transcriptional gene silencing in Drosophila cells. Nature. 2000;**404**(6775):293-296

[8] Ruby JG, Jan CH, Bartel DP. Intronic microRNA precursors that bypass Drosha processing. Nature. 2007;**448**(7149):83-86

[9] Yang JS, Lai EC. Alternative miRNA biogenesis pathways and the interpretation of core miRNA pathway mutants. Molecular Cell. 2011;**43**(6):892-903

[10] Tanzer A, Stadler PF. Molecular evolution of a microRNA cluster. Journal of Molecular Biology. 2004;**339**(2):327-335

[11] Yoda M, Kawamata T, Paroo Z, Ye X, Iwasaki S, Liu Q, et al. ATP-dependent human RISC assembly pathways. Nature Structural & Molecular Biology. 2010;**17**(1):17-23

[12] Meijer HA, Smith EM, Bushell M. Regulation of miRNA strand selection: Follow the leader? Biochemical Society Transactions. 2014;**42**(4):1135-1140

[13] Brennecke J, Aravin AA, Stark A, Dus M, Kellis M, Sachidanandam R, et al. Discrete small RNA-generating loci as master regulators of transposon activity in Drosophila. Cell. 2007;**128**(6):1089-1103

[14] Weick EM, Miska EA. piRNAs: From biogenesis to function. Development. 2014;**141**(18):3458-3471

[15] Vourekas A, Zheng Q, Alexiou P, Maragkakis M, Kirino Y, Gregory BD, et al. Mili and Miwi target RNA repertoire reveals piRNA biogenesis and function of Miwi in spermiogenesis. Nature Structural & Molecular Biology. 2012;**19**(8):773-781

[16] Ishizu H, Siomi H, Siomi MC. Biology of PIWI-interacting RNAs: New insights into biogenesis and function inside and outside of germlines. Genes & Development. 2012;**26**(21):2361-2373

[17] Friedman RC, Farh KK, Burge CB, Bartel DP. Most mammalian mRNAs are conserved targets of microRNAs. Genome Research. 2009;**19**(1):92-105

[18] Thomson T, Lin H. The biogenesis and function of PIWI proteins and piRNAs: Progress and prospect. Annual

Review of Cell and Developmental Biology. 2009;**25**:355-376

[19] Valadkhan S, Gunawardane LS. Role of small nuclear RNAs in eukaryotic gene expression. Essays in Biochemistry. 2013;**54**:79-90

[20] Brameier M, Herwig A, Reinhardt R, Walter L, Gruber J. Human box C/D snoRNAs with miRNA like functions: Expanding the range of regulatory RNAs. Nucleic Acids Research. 2011;**39**(2):675-686

[21] Watanabe T, Totoki Y, Toyoda A, Kaneda M, Kuramochi-Miyagawa S, Obata Y, et al. Endogenous siRNAs from naturally formed dsRNAs regulate transcripts in mouse oocytes. Nature. 2008;**453**(7194):539-543

[22] Ivanov P, Emara MM, Villen J, Gygi SP, Anderson P. Angiogenin-induced tRNA fragments inhibit translation initiation. Molecular Cell. 2011;**43**(4):613-623

[23] Wolin SL, Steitz JA. Genes for two small cytoplasmic Ro RNAs are adjacent and appear to be single-copy in the human genome. Cell. 1983;**32**(3):735-744

[24] Ullu E, Weiner AM. Human genes and pseudogenes for the 7SL RNA component of signal recognition particle. The EMBO Journal. 1984;**3**(13):3303-3310

[25] Parrott AM, Mathews MB. Novel rapidly evolving hominid RNAs bind nuclear factor 90 and display tissue-restricted distribution. Nucleic Acids Research. 2007;**35**(18):6249-6258

[26] Stadler PF, Chen JJ, Hackermuller J, Hoffmann S, Horn F, Khaitovich P, et al. Evolution of vault RNAs. Molecular Biology and Evolution. 2009;**26**(9):1975-1991

[27] Horwich MD, Li C, Matranga C, Vagin V, Farley G, Wang P, et al. The Drosophila RNA methyltransferase, DmHen1, modifies germline piRNAs and single-stranded siRNAs in RISC. Current Biology. 2007;**17**(14):1265-1272

[28] Lim SL, Qu ZP, Kortschak RD, Lawrence DM, Geoghegan J, Hempfling AL, et al. HENMT1 and piRNA stability are required for adult male germ cell transposon repression and to define the spermatogenic program in the mouse. PLoS Genetics. 2015;**11**(10):e1005620

[29] Czech B, Hannon GJ. One loop to rule them all: The ping-pong cycle and piRNA-guided silencing. Trends in Biochemical Sciences. 2016;**41**(4):324-337

[30] Grimson A, Srivastava M, Fahey B, Woodcroft BJ, Chiang HR, King N, et al. Early origins and evolution of microRNAs and Piwi-interacting RNAs in animals. Nature. 2008;**455**(7217):1193-1197

[31] Gunawardane LS, Saito K, Nishida KM, Miyoshi K, Kawamura Y, Nagami T, et al. A slicer-mediated mechanism for repeat-associated siRNA 5' end formation in Drosophila. Science. 2007;**315**(5818):1587-1590

[32] Kim VN, Han J, Siomi MC. Biogenesis of small RNAs in animals. Nature Reviews. Molecular Cell Biology. 2009;**10**(2):126-139

[33] Bartel DP. MicroRNAs: Target recognition and regulatory functions. Cell. 2009;**136**(2):215-233

[34] Hutvagner G, Simard MJ. Argonaute proteins: Key players in RNA silencing. Nature Reviews. Molecular Cell Biology. 2008;**9**(1):22-32

[35] Behm-Ansmant I, Rehwinkel J, Doerks T, Stark A, Bork P, Izaurralde E. mRNA degradation by miRNAs and GW182 requires both CCR4:NOT deadenylase and DCP1:DCP2 decapping

complexes. Genes & Development. 2006;**20**(14):1885-1898

[36] Meijer HA, Kong YW, Lu WT, Wilczynska A, Spriggs RV, Robinson SW, et al. Translational repression and eIF4A2 activity are critical for microRNA-mediated gene regulation. Science. 2013;**340**(6128):82-85

[37] Truesdell SS, Mortensen RD, Seo M, Schroeder JC, Lee JH, LeTonqueze O, et al. MicroRNA-mediated mRNA translation activation in quiescent cells and oocytes involves recruitment of a nuclear microRNP. Scientific Reports. 2012;**2**:842

[38] Nishi K, Nishi A, Nagasawa T, Ui-Tei K. Human TNRC6A is an argonaute-navigator protein for microRNA-mediated gene silencing in the nucleus. RNA. 2013;**19**(1):17-35

[39] Volpe TA, Kidner C, Hall IM, Teng G, Grewal SI, Martienssen RA. Regulation of heterochromatic silencing and histone H3 lysine-9 methylation by RNAi. Science. 2002;**297**(5588):1833-1837

[40] Benhamed M, Herbig U, Ye T, Dejean A, Bischof O. Senescence is an endogenous trigger for microRNA-directed transcriptional gene silencing in human cells. Nature Cell Biology. 2012;**14**(3):266-275

[41] Xiao M, Li J, Li W, Wang Y, Wu F, Xi Y, et al. MicroRNAs activate gene transcription epigenetically as an enhancer trigger. RNA Biology. 2017;**14**(10):1326-1334

[42] Allo M, Agirre E, Bessonov S, Bertucci P, Gomez Acuna L, Buggiano V, et al. Argonaute-1 binds transcriptional enhancers and controls constitutive and alternative splicing in human cells. Proceedings of the National Academy of Sciences of the United States of America. 2014;**111**(44):15622-15629

[43] Bottini S, Hamouda-Tekaya N, Mategot R, Zaragosi LE, Audebert S, Pisano S, et al. Post-transcriptional gene silencing mediated by microRNAs is controlled by nucleoplasmic Sfpq. Nature Communications. 2017;**8**(1):1189

[44] Iftikhar H, Carney GE. Evidence and potential in vivo functions for biofluid miRNAs: From expression profiling to functional testing: Potential roles of extracellular miRNAs as indicators of physiological change and as agents of intercellular information exchange. BioEssays. 2016;**38**(4):367-378

[45] Khurana JS, Theurkauf W. piRNAs, transposon silencing, and Drosophila germline development. The Journal of Cell Biology. 2010;**191**(5):905-913

[46] Sienski G, Donertas D, Brennecke J. Transcriptional silencing of transposons by Piwi and maelstrom and its impact on chromatin state and gene expression. Cell. 2012;**151**(5):964-980

[47] Grimaud C, Bantignies F, Pal-Bhadra M, Ghana P, Bhadra U, Cavalli G. RNAi components are required for nuclear clustering of polycomb group response elements. Cell. 2006;**124**(5):957-971

[48] Pal-Bhadra M, Leibovitch BA, Gandhi SG, Chikka MR, Bhadra U, Birchler JA, et al. Heterochromatic silencing and HP1 localization in Drosophila are dependent on the RNAi machinery. Science. 2004;**303**(5658):669-672

[49] Luteijn MJ, Ketting RF. PIWI-interacting RNAs: From generation to transgenerational epigenetics. Nature Reviews. Genetics. 2013;**14**(8):523-534

[50] Jones BC, Wood JG, Chang C, Tam AD, Franklin MJ, Siegel ER, et al. A somatic piRNA pathway in the Drosophila fat body ensures metabolic homeostasis and normal lifespan. Nature Communications. 2016;**7**:13856

[51] Moyano M, Stefani G. piRNA involvement in genome stability and human cancer. Journal of Hematology & Oncology. 2015;**8**:38

[52] Ross RJ, Weiner MM, Lin H. PIWI proteins and PIWI-interacting RNAs in the soma. Nature. 2014;**505**(7483):353-359

[53] Mestdagh P, Hartmann N, Baeriswyl L, Andreasen D, Bernard N, Chen C, et al. Evaluation of quantitative miRNA expression platforms in the microRNA quality control (miRQC) study. Nature Methods. 2014;**11**(8):809-815

[54] Wang Z, Gerstein M, Snyder M. RNA-Seq: A revolutionary tool for transcriptomics. Nature Reviews. Genetics. 2009;**10**(1):57-63

[55] Londin E, Loher P, Telonis AG, Quann K, Clark P, Jing Y, et al. Analysis of 13 cell types reveals evidence for the expression of numerous novel primate- and tissue-specific microRNAs. Proceedings of the National Academy of Sciences of the United States of America. 2015;**112**(10):E1106-E1115

[56] Martinez VD, Vucic EA, Thu KL, Hubaux R, Enfield KS, Pikor LA, et al. Unique somatic and malignant expression patterns implicate PIWI-interacting RNAs in cancer-type specific biology. Scientific Reports. 2015;**5**:10423

[57] Bracken CP, Scott HS, Goodall GJ. A network-biology perspective of microRNA function and dysfunction in cancer. Nature Reviews. Genetics. 2016;**17**(12):719-732

[58] Enfield KS, Pikor LA, Martinez VD, Lam WL. Mechanistic roles of noncoding RNAs in lung cancer biology and their clinical implications. Genetics Research International. 2012;**2012**:737416

[59] Vucic EA, Thu KL, Pikor LA, Enfield KS, Yee J, English JC, et al.

Smoking status impacts microRNA mediated prognosis and lung adenocarcinoma biology. BMC Cancer. 2014;**14**:778

[60] Calin GA, Croce CM. MicroRNA signatures in human cancers. Nature Reviews. Cancer. 2006;**6**(11):857-866

[61] Hammond SM. An overview of microRNAs. Advanced Drug Delivery Reviews. 2015;**87**:3-14

[62] Marshall EA, Sage AP, Ng KW, Martinez VD, Firmino NS, Bennewith KL, et al. Small non-coding RNA transcriptome of the NCI-60 cell line panel. Scientific Data. 2017;**4**:170157

[63] Minatel BC, Martinez VD, Ng KW, Sage AP, Tokar T, Marshall EA, et al. Large-scale discovery of previously undetected microRNAs specific to human liver. Human Genomics. 2018;**12**(1):16

[64] Sage AP, Minatel BC, Marshall EA, Martinez VD, Stewart GL, Enfield KSS, et al. Expanding the miRNA transcriptome of human kidney and renal cell carcinoma. International Journal of Genomics. 2018;**2018**:6972397

[65] Friedlander MR, Mackowiak SD, Li N, Chen W, Rajewsky N. miRDeep2 accurately identifies known and hundreds of novel microRNA genes in seven animal clades. Nucleic Acids Research. 2012;**40**(1):37-52

[66] Griffiths-Jones S, Saini HK, van Dongen S, Enright AJ. miRBase: Tools for microRNA genomics. Nucleic Acids Research. 2008;**36**(Database issue):D154-D158

[67] Mutz KO, Heilkenbrinker A, Lonne M, Walter JG, Stahl F. Transcriptome analysis using next-generation sequencing. Current Opinion in Biotechnology. 2013;**24**(1):22-30

[68] Peterson SM, Thompson JA, Ufkin ML, Sathyanarayana P, Liaw L, Congdon CB. Common features of microRNA target prediction tools. Frontiers in Genetics. 2014;5:23

[69] Ozata DM, Gainetdinov I, Zoch A, O'Carroll D, Zamore PD. PIWI-interacting RNAs: Small RNAs with big functions. Nature Reviews. Genetics. 2019;20:89-108

[70] Cox DN, Chao A, Lin H. Piwi encodes a nucleoplasmic factor whose activity modulates the number and division rate of germline stem cells. Development. 2000;127(3):503-514

[71] Krishnan P, Damaraju S. The challenges and opportunities in the clinical application of noncoding RNAs: The road map for miRNAs and piRNAs in cancer diagnostics and prognostics. International Journal of Genomics. 2018;2018:5848046

[72] Zuo L, Wang Z, Tan Y, Chen X, Luo X. piRNAs and their functions in the brain. International Journal of Human Genetics. 2016;16(1-2):53-60

[73] Lee EJ, Banerjee S, Zhou H, Jammalamadaka A, Arcila M, Manjunath BS, et al. Identification of piRNAs in the central nervous system. RNA. 2011;17(6):1090-1099

[74] Girard A, Sachidanandam R, Hannon GJ, Carmell MA. A germline-specific class of small RNAs binds mammalian Piwi proteins. Nature. 2006;442(7099):199-202

[75] Keam SP, Young PE, McCorkindale AL, Dang TH, Clancy JL, Humphreys DT, et al. The human Piwi protein Hiwi2 associates with tRNA-derived piRNAs in somatic cells. Nucleic Acids Research. 2014;42(14):8984-8995

[76] Wang J, Zhang P, Lu Y, Li Y, Zheng Y, Kan Y, et al. piRBase: A comprehensive database of piRNA sequences. Nucleic Acids Research. 2019;47(D1):D175-D180

[77] Sai Lakshmi S, Agrawal S. piRNABank: A web resource on classified and clustered Piwi-interacting RNAs. Nucleic Acids Research. 2008;36(Database issue):D173-D177

[78] Balatti V, Nigita G, Veneziano D, Drusco A, Stein GS, Messier TL, et al. tsRNA signatures in cancer. Proceedings of the National Academy of Sciences of the United States of America. 2017;114(30):8071-8076

[79] Watanabe T, Lin H. Posttranscriptional regulation of gene expression by Piwi proteins and piRNAs. Molecular Cell. 2014;56(1):18-27

[80] Batista PJ, Ruby JG, Claycomb JM, Chiang R, Fahlgren N, Kasschau KD, et al. PRG-1 and 21U-RNAs interact to form the piRNA complex required for fertility in C. Elegans. Molecular Cell. 2008;31(1):67-78

[81] Toombs JA, Sytnikova YA, Chirn GW, Ang I, Lau NC, Blower MD. Xenopus Piwi proteins interact with a broad proportion of the oocyte transcriptome. RNA. 2017;23(4):504-520

[82] Zhang D, Tu S, Stubna M, Wu WS, Huang WC, Weng Z, et al. The piRNA targeting rules and the resistance to piRNA silencing in endogenous genes. Science. 2018;359(6375):587-592

[83] Enright AJ, John B, Gaul U, Tuschl T, Sander C, Marks DS. MicroRNA targets in Drosophila. Genome Biology. 2003;5(1):R1

[84] Hashim A, Rizzo F, Marchese G, Ravo M, Tarallo R, Nassa G, et al. RNA sequencing identifies specific PIWI-interacting small non-coding RNA expression patterns in breast cancer. Oncotarget. 2014;5(20):9901-9910

[85] Yang Y, Zhang X, Song D, Wei J. Piwil2 modulates the invasion and metastasis of prostate cancer by regulating the expression of matrix metalloproteinase-9 and epithelial-mesenchymal transitions. Oncology Letters. 2015;**10**(3):1735-1740

[86] Schudrowitz N, Takagi S, Wessel GM, Yajima M. Germline factor DDX4 functions in blood-derived cancer cell phenotypes. Cancer Science. 2017;**108**(8):1612-1619

[87] Mei Y, Wang Y, Kumari P, Shetty AC, Clark D, Gable T, et al. A piRNA-like small RNA interacts with and modulates p-ERM proteins in human somatic cells. Nature Communications. 2015;**6**:7316

[88] Firmino N, Martinez VD, Rowbotham DA, Enfield KSS, Bennewith KL, Lam WL. HPV status is associated with altered PIWI-interacting RNA expression pattern in head and neck cancer. Oral Oncology. 2016;**55**:43-48

[89] Krishnan AR, Korrapati A, Zou AE, Qu Y, Wang XQ, Califano JA, et al. Smoking status regulates a novel panel of PIWI-interacting RNAs in head and neck squamous cell carcinoma. Oral Oncology. 2017;**65**:68-75

[90] Nogueira Jorge NA, Wajnberg G, Ferreira CG, de Sa Carvalho B, Passetti F. snoRNA and piRNA expression levels modified by tobacco use in women with lung adenocarcinoma. PLoS One. 2017;**12**(8):e0183410

[91] Weng W, Liu N, Toiyama Y, Kusunoki M, Nagasaka T, Fujiwara T, et al. Novel evidence for a PIWI-interacting RNA (piRNA) as an oncogenic mediator of disease progression, and a potential prognostic biomarker in colorectal cancer. Molecular Cancer. 2018;**17**(1):16

[92] Li Y, Wu X, Gao H, Jin JM, Li AX, Kim YS, et al. Piwi-interacting RNAs (piRNAs) are Dysregulated in renal cell carcinoma and associated with tumor metastasis and cancer-specific survival. Molecular Medicine. 2015;**21**:381-388

[93] Huang G, Hu H, Xue X, Shen S, Gao E, Guo G, et al. Altered expression of piRNAs and their relation with clinicopathologic features of breast cancer. Clinical & Translational Oncology. 2013;**15**(7):563-568

[94] Cheng J, Guo JM, Xiao BX, Miao Y, Jiang Z, Zhou H, et al. piRNA, the new non-coding RNA, is aberrantly expressed in human cancer cells. Clinica Chimica Acta. 2011;**412**(17-18):1621-1625

[95] Yan H, Wu QL, Sun CY, Ai LS, Deng J, Zhang L, et al. piRNA-823 contributes to tumorigenesis by regulating de novo DNA methylation and angiogenesis in multiple myeloma. Leukemia. 2015;**29**(1):196-206

[96] Das B, Roy J, Jain N, Mallick B. Tumor suppressive activity of PIWI-interacting RNA in human fibrosarcoma mediated through repression of RRM2. Molecular Carcinogenesis. 2018;1-14

[97] Wang QE, Han C, Milum K, Wani AA. Stem cell protein Piwil2 modulates chromatin modifications upon cisplatin treatment. Mutation Research. 2011;**708**(1-2):59-68

[98] Wang Y, Gable T, Ma MZ, Clark D, Zhao J, Zhang Y, et al. A piRNA-like small RNA induces chemoresistance to cisplatin-based therapy by inhibiting apoptosis in lung squamous cell carcinoma. Molecular Therapy. Nucleic Acids. 2017;**6**:269-278

[99] Balaratnam S, West N, Basu S. A piRNA utilizes HILI and HIWI2 mediated pathway to down-regulate ferritin heavy chain 1 mRNA in human somatic cells. Nucleic Acids Research. 2018;**46**(20):10635-10648

[100] Lithwick-Yanai G, Dromi N, Shtabsky A, Morgenstern S, Strenov Y,

Feinmesser M, et al. Multicentre validation of a microRNA-based assay for diagnosing indeterminate thyroid nodules utilising fine needle aspirate smears. Journal of Clinical Pathology. 2017;**70**(6):500-507

[101] Martinez VD, Enfield KS, Rowbotham DA, Lam WL. An atlas of gastric PIWI-interacting RNA transcriptomes and their utility for identifying signatures of gastric cancer recurrence. Gastric Cancer. 2016;**19**(2):660-665

[102] Xu R, Rai A, Chen M, Suwakulsiri W, Greening DW, Simpson RJ. Extracellular vesicles in cancer—Implications for future improvements in cancer care. Nature Reviews. Clinical Oncology. 2018;**15**(10):617-638

[103] Anfossi S, Babayan A, Pantel K, Calin GA. Clinical utility of circulating non-coding RNAs—An update. Nature Reviews. Clinical Oncology. 2018;**15**(9):541-563

[104] Umu SU, Langseth H, Bucher-Johannessen C, Fromm B, Keller A, Meese E, et al. A comprehensive profile of circulating RNAs in human serum. RNA Biology. 2018;**15**(2):242-250

[105] Ren J, Zhou Q, Li H, Li J, Pang L, Su L, et al. Characterization of exosomal RNAs derived from human gastric cancer cells by deep sequencing. Tumour Biology. 2017;**39**(4):1010428317695012

[106] Yuan T, Huang X, Woodcock M, Du M, Dittmar R, Wang Y, et al. Plasma extracellular RNA profiles in healthy and cancer patients. Scientific Reports. 2016;**6**:19413

[107] Kleivi Sahlberg K, Bottai G, Naume B, Burwinkel B, Calin GA, Borresen-Dale AL, et al. A serum microRNA signature predicts tumor relapse and survival in triple-negative breast cancer patients. Clinical Cancer Research. 2015;**21**(5):1207-1214

[108] Vychytilova-Faltejskova P, Stitkovcova K, Radova L, Sachlova M, Kosarova Z, Slaba K, et al. Circulating PIWI-interacting RNAs piR-5937 and piR-28876 are promising diagnostic biomarkers of colon cancer. Cancer Epidemiology, Biomarkers & Prevention. 2018;**27**(9):1019-1028

Chapter 3

The Role of Long Noncoding RNAs in Gene Expression Regulation

Zhijin Li, Weiling Zhao, Maode Wang and Xiaobo Zhou

Abstract

Accumulating evidence highlights that noncoding RNAs, especially the long noncoding RNAs (lncRNAs), are critical regulators of gene expression in development, differentiation, and human diseases, such as cancers and heart diseases. The regulatory mechanisms of lncRNAs have been categorized into four major archetypes: signals, decoys, scaffolds, and guides. Increasing evidence points that lncRNAs are able to regulate almost every cellular process by their binding to proteins, mRNAs, miRNA, and/or DNAs. In this review, we present the recent research advances about the regulatory mechanisms of lncRNA in gene expression at various levels, including pretranscription, transcription regulation, and posttranscription regulation. We also introduce the interaction between lncRNA and DNA, RNA and protein, and the bioinformatics applications on lncRNA research.

Keywords: long noncoding RNAs, gene regulation, lncRNA binding, bioinformatics

1. Introduction

It was estimated that there are approximately 20,500 protein coding genes that account for 2% of the genome [1], and another 98% of the genome were considered as "DNA junks" previously due to their disability in coding proteins. The application of high-throughput next generation sequencing (NGS) technology has changed our view of the genome, about 90% of the human genome can be transcribed into RNA transcripts [2–5]. Except the small portion of transcripts encoding for proteins, the majority of RNA transcripts in the type have been grouped into noncoding RNAs (ncRNAs), including transfer RNAs (tRNAs), ribosomal RNAs (rRNAs), small ncRNAs such as micro RNAs (miRNAs), small interfering RNAs (siRNAs), small nuclear RNAs (snRNA), circular RNA, as well as long ncRNAs (lncRNAs). The rRNA and tRNA are two basic ant most abundant RNAs that play important roles in mRNA translation. The miRNAs are short single strand RNAs of 20–22 base with the role of promoting mRNA degradation. SiRNA is a class of double strand RNA with a length of 20–25 base pairs, which interferes target gene expression by degrading mRNA or preventing translation. The snRNA, with an average length of 150 base, is a class of small RNA located in nucleus speckles. The primary function of snRNA is in the processing of pre-mRNA splicing. Circular RNAs is a very special class of ncRNA. The 3′ and 5′ ends of the circular RNA join together to form a covalently closed continuous loop. The

IntechOpen

function of the circular RNA is not clear. LncRNAs are defined as the noncoding linear transcripts longer than 200 nucleotides, which have different features with other ncRNA listed above. In general, they share common characteristics with mRNAs. The majority of LncRNAs are usually transcribed by RNA polymerase II, capped at 5′ end, and spliced; most of them are also polyadenylated at the 3′ end and have promoter regions. Compared to the protein coding gene mRNA, lncRNAs lack of open reading frame (ORF), contain fewer exons (~2.8 exons in lncRNAs compared to 11 exons for protein coding gene), are expressed in low abundance and more tissue-specific [6]. Some of them have no polyadenylation tails. The lncRNAs account for the major class of the ncRNAs in the gnome. There are ~30,000 high-confidence transcripts of lncRNAs in human according to GENCODE reference genome annotation [7], and more and more new lncRNAs are coming into the light. The database LNCipedia has collected 127,802 transcripts from 56,946 long noncoding genes in human [8, 9]. Many of the ncRNAs have been confirmed as playing crucial regulatory roles in diverse biological processes and tumorigenesis. Increasing evidence indicates that lncRNAs play important roles in various cellular processes, such as DNA repair [10], proliferation [11], epithelial-mesenchymal transition (EMT) [12] by regulating various aspects of the related gene expression. LncRNAs have been associated with various diseases [13–16] and identified as potential biomarkers in some diseases, such as cancers, cardiovascular diseases, nervous system diseases, etc. [17–19]. LncRNAs could regulate gene expression by serving as molecular signals, guides, decoys and/or scaffolds [20]. In this review, we will present the recent research advances about the regulatory mechanisms of lncRNAs in gene expression at various levels, including pretranscription, transcription regulation, and post transcription regulation. We will also discuss the interaction between lncRNA and DNA, RNA and protein, as well as the applications of bioinformatics in lncRNA-related research.

2. The role of lncRNA in pretranscription regulation

Gene expression is regulated at many levels, such as epigenetic, transcriptional, post-transcriptional, translational, and post-translational. In order to be transcribed, changes in the chromatin structure of a gene must take place to make the chromatin open to polymerases and transcriptional factors (TFs). Modification on chromatin DNA and histones affects gene accessibility and is associated with distinct transcription states. For example, H3 hyperacetylation or methylation at lysine 4 often makes the gene easily accessible, thereby actively transcribed. In contrast, histone methylation at lysine 9 results the assembly of compact or closed chromatin around the DNA, leading to transcription silence. A number of epigenetic control factors have been identified to modify histones. Some of them can facilitate transcriptional activation, such as p300/CBP, Esa1, and TAF1, and others participate in transcriptional silencing, such as EZH2 and Ubc9. However, the majority of epigenetic factors, such as DNA methyltransferases/demethylases and histone modification enzymes may not efficiently recognize specific DNA sequences. Emerging studies show that lncRNAs can act as signals, guides or scaffolds at chromatin level to regulate gene expression [21–23]. LncRNAs have been reported to participate in the methylation processes. For example, Wang et al. found that lncRNA Dum (developmental pluripotency-associated 2 (Dppa2) Upstream binding Muscle lncRNA) regulated DPPa2 expression by affecting DNA methylation [24]. Dnmt proteins are known as DNA methyltransferases. Dum promoted DNA methylation of Dppa2 promoter by recruiting Dnmt1, Dnmt3a, and Dnmt3b to its promoter site, thereby silencing Dppa2 expression in cis and stimulating myogenic differentiation. Studies show that lncRNA HOTAIR (Hox transcript antisense intergenic RNA), transcribed from chromosome 12, can coordinate histone modification by binding to histone modifiers [25, 26]. Rinn et al. found that knock-down of HOTAIR led to transcriptional activation of HOXD locus genes present in the chromosome 2 and HOTAIR binding is required to guide polycomb repressive complex 2 (PRC2) to the HOXD locus [26]. PRC2 is epigenetic factor and can catalyze methylation on lysine 27 of histone H3 (H3K27). PRC2 and LSD1 (lysine-specific demethylase 1) bind to the 5′ and 3′ domains of HOTAIR, respectively. The HOTAIR-PRC2-LSD1 complex then targets the HOXD locus on the chromosome 2, silencing the genes involved in the suppression of metastasis. LncRNA HOTTIP (HOXA transcript at the distal tip) binds to and targets WDR5-MLL complexes to the 5′ HOXA locus, mediating the transcriptional activation of HOXA via driving H3K4 methylation [27]. LncRNA Evf-2 interacts with methy-CpG binding protein 2 (MECP2), inhibiting the methylation at DLX5/6 enhancer [28]. Similarly, LncRNA GClnc1 (gastric cancer–associated lncRNA 1) promotes gastric carcinogenesis by acting as a modular scaffold of WDR5 and KAT2A complexes to specify the histone modification pattern on superoxide dismutase 2 [29]. Zhao et al. showed that lncRNA PAPAS (promoter and pre-rRNA antisense) guided CHD4/NuRD (nucleosome remodeling and deacetylation) to the rDNA promoter by forming a DNA-RNA triplex structure at the enhancer region of rDNA [30]. Other studies have also explored the role of lncRNAs in epigenetic regulation of transcription [31, 32].

3. The role of lncRNA in transcription regulation

Transcription begins with the binding of RNA polymerase II to the promoter region of a gene with the support of general transcription factors (GTFs). Other transcription factors (TFs) bind to the enhancer region accelerate transcription. The transcription is terminated when the polymerase meets to the terminator. LncRNAs can regulate gene expression by direct binding with TFs or PNA Pol II, or interfering the binding polymerase with promotor. For example, lncMyoD is an lncRNA activated by myogenic differentiation (MyoD) during myogenesis. LncMyoD can directly binds to IGF2-mRNA-binding protein 2 (IMP2) and negatively regulates IMP2-mediated translation of proliferation genes such as N-Ras and c-Myc, which create a permissive state for differentiation [33]. lncRNA Gas5 (growth arrest-specific 5) attenuates some of GR positive related gene expression by binding to glucose receptors (GR) [24]. LncHIFCAR (long noncoding HIF-1α co-activating RNA) level is upregulated in oral carcinoma. Shiih et al. found that LncHIFCAR acted as a HIF-1α co-activator driving oral cancer progression [34]. LncHIFCAR formed a complex with HIF-1α via directly binding and facilitates the recruitment of HIF-1α and p300 cofactor to the target promoters. In addition, lncRNAs can guide RNA polymerase II to bind to the promoter of specific genes. Miao et al. found that lncRNA LEENE guided and facilitated the recruitment of RNA Pol II to the eNOS promoter to upregulate eNOS RNA transcription [35]. In addition, recent studies indicated that lncRNA gene promoter could compete for enhancer with protein coding gene promoter. Enhancer is the cis-acting DNA sequence that can enhance the transcription of an associated gene, when bound by specific transcription factors. Cho et al. found that the lncRNA PVT1 promoter has a tumor-suppressor function that is independent of PVT1 gene [36]. The promoter of lncRNA PVT1 competes with the Myc promoter for engagement to four intragenic enhancers, thereby inhibiting the expression of Myc gene.

4. lncRNA on posttranscription regulation

After transcription, the pre-mRNAs are regulated by various RNA-binding proteins (RBPs). The pre-mRNAs are capped, polyadenylated, spliced, edited and transferred from nucleus to cytoplasm. The stability of mRNA is also an important aspect for translation. There are evidence showing the role of lncRNAs in mRNA splicing, editing, transporting, mRNA stability, and mRNA translation. In addition, lncRNAs can regulate mRNA expression indirectly by acting as competing endogenous RNAs.

4.1 lncRNA and alternative splicing

Alternative splicing is a regulatory process during gene expression that enables a single gene coding for multiple proteins. Recent studies indicate that lncRNA can regulate alternative splicing through two main mechanisms. LncRNAs can interact with specific splicing factors or form RNA-RNA duplexes with pre-mRNAs. SR (splicing factor) proteins, such as SRSF1, are a conserved family of proteins involved in RNA splicing regulation in a concentration- and phosphorylation-dependent manner. MALAT1 is a highly conserved lncRNA among mammals and predominantly localizes to nuclear speckles. Tripathi et al. [37] showed that MALAT1 acts as a molecular sponge to titrate the cellular pool of SR splicing factors, affecting the distribution of splicing factors in nuclear speckles where the alternative splicing occurs and ultimately controlling alternative splicing. The 5' region of MALAT1 can also bind to the serine/arginine domain of SRSF1 and regulates its cellular levels of the phosphorylated forms. SORL1 (Sorting Protein-Related Receptor Containing LDLR Class A Repeats), a sorting receptor for amyloid precursor protein (APP), can interact with amyloid APP and affect its transport and process in brain. Downregulation of SORL1 expression increases APP secretion and subsequently Aβ formation. LncRNA 51A, an antisense mapping to the intron 1 of the SORL1 gene, masked canonical splicing sites by pairing with SORL1 pre-mRNA, driving a splicing shift of SORL1 from the canonical long protein variant A to an alternatively spliced protein form B [38].

4.2 The regulation of lncRNA on mRNA stability

Different mRNAs have different lifespans, even in a single cell. The greater the stability of an mRNA molecule is, the more proteins may be produced by the mRNA molecule. The steady-state level of a mRNA is determined by the rate of synthesis and degradation. Modulation of mRNA degradation is an important control point in gene expression to regulate protein synthesis in response to physiological needs and environmental signals. Studies have shown that the role of lncRNA in the regulation of mRNA stability. For example, Cao et al. found that lncRNA LAST (LncRNA-Assisted Stabilization of Transcripts) acted as a mRNA stabilizer by cooperating with CNBP (CCHC-type zinc finger nucleic acid binding protein) to promote Cyclin D1 mRNA stability [39]. Antisense lncRNAs are transcripts emerging from the opposite strand of a coding-RNA region. β-site amyloid precursor protein cleaving enzyme (BACE1) is involved in the production of the amyloid-β (Aβ) peptides that form plaques in the brains of individuals with AD. BACE1-AS expression is elevated in the brain of Alzheimer mouse model. Faghihi et al. found that BACE1-AS increased the stability of BACE1 mRNA and upregulated the BACE1 protein by forming RNA duplex with BACE1 mRNA, which masked the binding site for miR-485-5p and thereby increase the BACE1 mRNA stability [40, 41]. Matsui et al. found that iNOS antisense transcript stabilized iNOS mRNA through interaction with AU-rich element-binding HuR protein [42]. lncRNAs can also reduce the stability of mRNA by making the transcript prone to degradation. aHIF is a natural antisense transcript of hypoxia-inducible factor 1alpha (HIF-1α). Rossignol et al. reported that aHIF could expose AU-riches elements present in the HIF-1α mRNA 3' UTR, thus increasing the degradation speed of HIF-1a mRNA [43].

4.3 lncRNA and protein stability

LncRNA can also directly interact with proteins and regulate their stability by retarding protein ubiquitination and degeneration. Androgen receptor (AR) is a critical risk factor in castration-resistant prostate cancer. Zhang et al. shown that lncRNA HOTAIR bound to AR protein to block AR interaction with E3 ubiquitin ligase MDM2, thereby preventing AR ubiquitination and AR protein degradation [44]. Liu et al. identified lncRNA MT1JP as a critical factor in restraining cell transformation by modulating p53 translation through binding and stabilizing the RNA binding protein TIAR [45]. LincRNA-p21 is a hypoxia-responsive lncRNA. LncRNA-p21 can bind to HIF-1 at its VHL binging region and attenuate VHL-mediated HIF-1α ubiquitination, leading to HIF-1α accumulation [46].

4.4 lncRNA regulates protein translation

Transcription and translation are two main stages in gene expression. In translation, the ribosomal preinitiation complex, consisting of eukaryotic initiation factors (eIFs) and ribosomes, is positioned the start codon of the target RNA. With the help of tRNA, the mRNA is decoded to produce peptide chains. It has been reported that lncRNAs participate in protein translation by interaction with rRNA, ribosome or eIFs. Li et al. reported that a nucleolar-specific lncRNA, LoNA reduced rRNA production and ribosome biosynthesis [47]. The 5' region of LoNA bound to and sequestered nucleolin to suppress rRNA transcription and the 3' end recruited and diminishes fibrillarin activity to reduce rRNA methylation [47]. Tran et al. found that lncRNA AS-RBM15, the antisense of RNA binding motif protein 15, overlapped with the 5' UTR of RBM15. As-RBM15 enhanced RBM15 protein translation via incorporation into the RBM15 mRNA-containing polyribosome in a CAP-dependent manner [48]. The antisense of UCHL1 binds the 5' UTR of UCHL1 mRNA to active polysomes for UCHL1 translation [49]. LncRNA Gas5 (growth arrest specific 5) has been reported to interact and cooperate with eIF4E to regulate c-MYC translation [50].

4.5 lncRNAs act as microRNA sponges

Micro RNAs (miRNAs), short ncRNAs, can bind to the complementary regions of mRNAs to post-translationally regulate the expression of target genes. The subcellular localization of lncRNAs is associated with their functions. Studies have shown that lncRNAs can act as miRNA sponges to inhibit the binding of miRNAs to their mRNA targets, thereby stabilizing the target mRNAs and regulating the corresponding protein expression [51]. Hu et al. found that p53-responding lncRNA GUARDIN is important for maintaining genomic integrity under exogenous genotoxic stress. GUARDIN contains eight regions complementary to the 'seed' region of miR-23a. Telomeric repeat-binding factor-2 (TRF2), a critical component of the shelterin complex, is one of the targets of miR-23a. GUARDIN maintained the expression of TRF2 by sequestering miR-23a. Zhou et al. observed that lncRNA H19 acted as a sponge for the miRNAs miR-200b/c and Let-7b to promote an epithelial or mesenchymal switch in tumor cells [52]. In the epithelial-like tumor cells, H19 inhibited the migration-related protein ARF by sequestering miR-200b/c. In contrast, H19 activated ARF by sequestering Let-7b in the mesenchymal-like tumor cells. H19 stimulated HMGA2-mediated EMT by sequestering Let-7 to promote pancreatic ductal adenocarcinoma cell invasion and migration [52, 53].

4.6 lncRNA sequesters proteins

LncRNA can act as protein molecular decoy by binding and sequestering proteins, thereby inhibiting their functions [54]. Lee et al. identified a lncRNA named noncoding RNA activated by DNA damage (NORAD) [55] and found that NORAD played an important role in maintaining genomic stability by binding and sequestering PUMILIO proteins. In the absence of NORAD, PUMILIO proteins drove chromosomal instability by acting as negative regulators of gene expression involved in DNA damage repair and mitosis. S-adenosyl-L-homocysteine hydrolase (SAHH) is the only mammalian enzyme capable of catalyzing the hydrolysis of S-adenosyl-L-homocysteine (SAH), which is an inhibitor of S-adenosylmethionine (SAM)-dependent methyltransferases. Zhou et al. reported that lncRNA H19 bound to SAHH and suppressed its enzymatic activity, leading to an increased accumulation of SAH [56]. lncRNA Gas5 is induced by stress like starvation. Glucocorticoid receptor (GR) plays important role in regulating genes associated with metabolism, development and immune response. Kino et al. showed that lncRNA Gas5 bound to the DNA-binding domain of glucocorticoid receptor (GR), thereby, inhibiting the ability of GR to regulate the related gene expression [57].

5. The lncRNA interaction with other molecules

As shown above, lncRNAs regulate gene expression at pretranscriptional, transcriptional and posttranscriptional levels by interacting with DNAs, mRNAs, miRNAs, and proteins. Here we will give a brief introduction of the interactions of lncRNA with other molecules.

5.1 lncRNA-DNA

LncRNAs regulate gene expression through various complicated mechanisms, one of the them is binding to the DNA or forming RNA-dsDNA triplexes by targeting specific DNA sequences. The lncRNA as a third strand can inserted into the major groove of the DNA duplex by Hoogsteen hydrogen binding [58]. The Hoogsteen hydrogen binding by a third strand is usually weaker than the Watson-Crick hydrogen bonding. Studies from Roberts et al. indicate RNA may form more stable triplexes than their DNA counterparts [59]. Various methods have been used to investigate the interaction of lncRNA and DNA. The formation of lncRNA DHFR and dsDNA triplex was demonstrated using electrophoresis mobility shift assay [60] and the binding of lncRNA Fendrr to dsDNA was determined by *in vitro* pull-down experiments [61, 62]. High throughput methods are also applied to investigate the genomic binding sites of lncRNAs, such as capture hybridization analysis of RNA targets sequencing (CHART-seq) [63]. Although the mechanism of RNA-dsDNA triplexes formation is still not well illustrated, it is clear that the lncRNA-DNA interaction offers a potent mechanism for gene regulation. LncRNAs can bind DNAs acting as scaffolds for introducing proteins into the gene loci. When the proteins introduced by lncRNAs are methylation–related enzymes, these enzymes can induce promotor CpG island methylation or demethylation (**Figure 1A**). When the proteins imported by lncRNAs are histone modifier enzymes (**Figure 1A**), histone modifications can result gene expression, transcriptional silencing, or DNA

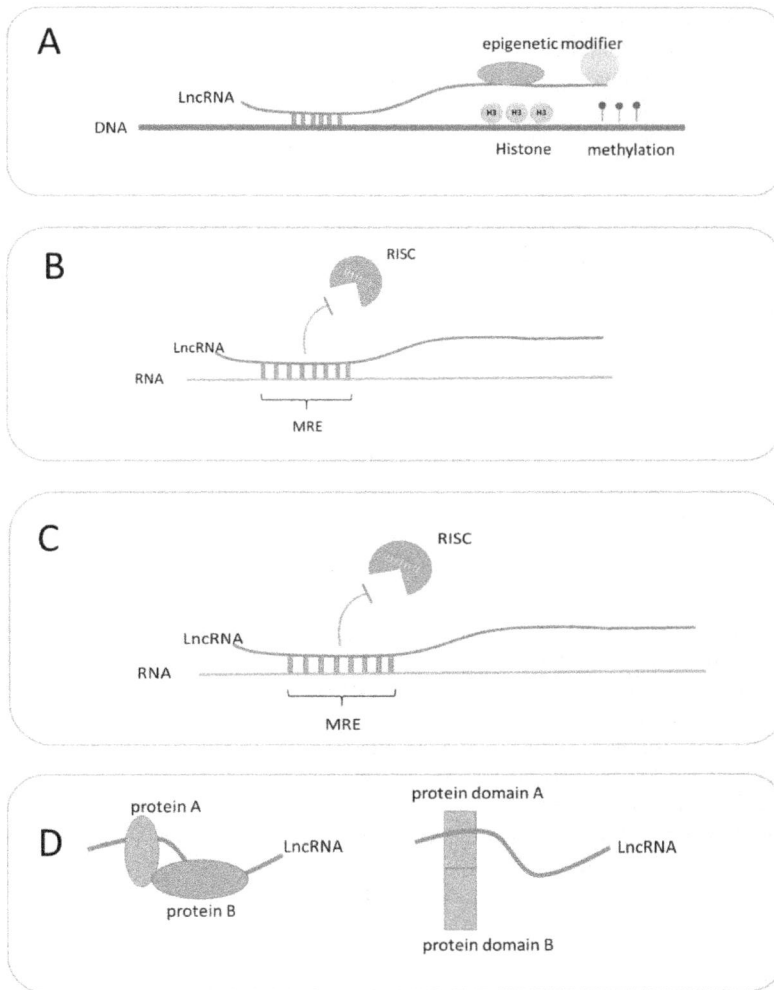

Figure 1.
The mechanisms of lncRNA regulating gene expression by interacting with other molecule. (A) lncRNA acting as scaffold binds to chromatin and epigenetic modifier, guide the epigenetic modifier to gene promotor. (B) lncRNA acting as miRNA sponges attenuates the miRNA' effect on downregulating mRNA expression. (C) lncRNA can bind to RNA' special region such as miRNA response element, thus masking the region. (D) lncRNA can act as scaffold for two or more protein, these proteins will act coordinately or act as a complex (left). lncRNA can bind to protein, the bonded protein domain may change its function (right).

repair and genomic imprinting. LncRNA can regulate either neighboring (cis) or distal (trans) protein coding genes. LncRNAs derived from one chromatin can bind to another chromatin, such as LncRNA HOTAIR, which is transcribed from the HOXC locus on the chromatin 12 and represses transcription in trans across 40 kb of the HOXD locus [26].

5.2 lncRNA-miRNA

The competitive endogenous RNA (ceRNA) hypothesis proposes that RNA transcripts, including both coding and noncoding RNAs, compete for post-translational regulation with shared miRNA binding sites (i.e. miRNA response elements) [64]. Cytoplasmic lncRNA can act as a molecular sponge of miRNA to regulate the rate of translation and degradation of mRNA (**Figure 1B**). RNA interference is a power-ful mechanism of gene silence and mediated by RNA-induced silencing complexes (RISC). RICS is ribonucleoprotein complex, which incorporates on strand of a single-stranded RNA fragment, such as miRNA [65]. Once a mRNA is transcribed and exported to the cytoplasm, it can be targeted by the RISC, resulting in the accel-erated degradation of the mRNA, or blocked translation. LncRNAs with miRNA response element can compete for miRNA targeting and binding to RISC, leading to sequestration of the microRNA-RISC and preventing RISC-mediated degradation of mRNAs and increasing mRNA expression. Using AGO-CLIP-seq high throughout method, thousands of miRNA-target interaction are estimated [66, 67]. We have shown studies that lncRNAs act as miRNA spongers above. Except lncRNAs, mRNA, circular RNAs and pseudogenes can also act s as the ceRNA. The most widely used miRNA target prediction rule is the 6-nucleotide interactions between 5' ends of the microRNA which is called "seed region" [68]. Note that one microRNA can binds to hundreds of RNAs and one RNA molecule may also bind to diverse microRNA with different affinity, which is difficult to quantify.

5.3 lncRNA-mRNA

As described above, lncRNAs are able to regulate pre-mRNA splicing and mRNA stability. Some antisense lncRNAs can bind to the homologous mRNA at the splice site, thereby masking the splice site and blocking spliceosome assembly [69]. LncRNAs can also mask miRNA target sites of an mRNA by binding to the mRNA at the miRNA response elements (**Figure 1C**), resulting in elevated stabil-ity and expression of the mRNA [40]. LncRNAs could bind to protein and mRNA simultaneously. Gong et al. reported that lncRNAs bound to the Alu region at the 3' UTR of mRNA and the looped lncRNAs bound to STAU1 protein (Double-Stranded RNA-Binding Protein Staufen Homolog 1), leading to the activation of the Staufen-mediated decay pathway [70]. Recently, computational and experimental methods have been developed to determine RNA–RNA interaction. For example, Sharma et al. [71] developed a high throughput sequencing method, named LIGation of interacting RNA followed by high-throughput sequencing" (LIGR-seq), to reveal a remarkable landscape of RNA-RNA interactions involving the major classes of ncRNA and mRNA. Nguyen developed MARIO (Mapping RNA interactome in vivo) [72] approach to map tens of thousands of endogenous RNA-RNA interactions.

5.4 lncRNA-protein

There is no double that RNA-protein interactions play a crucial role in fundamen-tal cellular processes. LncRNAs can function as protein decoys recruiting or seques-ter proteins, or act as scaffolds linking different proteins, which may act coordinately or act as a complex (**Figure 1D** left). Several models have been established to under-stand how an lncRNA regulates gene expression by protein binding. LncRNAs are able to recruit chromatin modifier to achieve chromatin modification [73]. LncRNA can bind and stabilize a protein by masking its ubiquitination site, inducing the accumulation of the target protein [44]. lncRNA can bind to protein, the bonded domain may change its function (**Figure 1D** right) [74]. LncRNAs can bind to TFs to mask their DNA-binding sequences or stabilize TFs [33]. LncRNAs are also able to bind to functional enzymes to inhibit their activities [33], resulting elevated levels of substrate proteins. The high throughput experimental methods, such as CLIP-seq and RIP-seq, have been used to study RNA-protein interactions [74].

5.5 The lncRNA location and its role

Most of lncRNAs are located exclusively in the nucleus, but some of them are located in the cytoplasm or in both nucleus and cytoplasm. Increasing evidence reveals that RNA subcellular location is a very important feature in understanding lncRNA functions. The nuclear function of lncRNAs are apt to regulate gene expression *in cis* or *in trans*. In the nucleus, a lncRNA can accumulate at its transcription site and recruit transcription factors or chromatin modifiers. LncRNAs in the nucleus also can regulate gene expression in trans by binding to a remote genome sites. In addition, the effect of lncRNA on alternative splicing usually occurs in the nucleus. The lncRNAs exported to cytoplasm intend to interfere translation or sequester proteins/miRNA. Currently, the subcellular locations of known lncRNAs are mainly determined by biological experiments. Most recently, Zhang et al. built a web-accessible database (RNALocate) to provide a high-quality RNA subcellular localization resource and facilitate future researches on RNA functions or structures based on the experimental data [75]. Su et al. developed a sequence-based bioinformatics tool (iLoc-lncRNA) to annotate and predict the subcellular locations of lncRNAs by binomial distribution of the 8-tuple nucleotide signatures into the general pseudo K-tuple nucleotide composition [76].

6. The application of bioinformatics in lncRNA studies

The research on LncRNAs research has increased rapidly in recent years. The bioinformaticians have developed various approaches for identification of lncRNA from the genome and transcriptome data, prediction of lncRNA structures, investigation of lncRNA functions and construction of lnRNA-associated regulatory networks. LncRNA databases have been established from some giant studies or by integrating different studies. The association analyses based methods, such as gene set enrichment analysis (GSEA) and weighted gene co-expression network analysis (WGCNA) make it easier for biologists to research the lncRNA. As described above, lncRNA can bind with single or multiple different types of molecules to regulate gene expression in the different level directly or indirectly. Therefore, the databases and tools are important for investigating lncRNA bindings with other molecules. The binding pattern is usually determined by the molecular sequences (nucleotide or amino acid) and the structures. Accumulated high throughput experimental methods have been developed for the identification of the lncRNA-DNA, lncRNA-RNA, and lncRNA-protein bindings. Based on these existing data, bioinformatics approaches, such as deep learning, can be used to identify the binding rules, which can be used to predict the potential molecule that could bind to given lncRNA based on the DNA/RNA sequences and/or structure. Note that the bioinformatics tools are useful, but one also should keep in mind that the prediction and associated analysis is a good screening process. Validation of the predicted results with experimental methods are required. Here, we briefly reviewed the bioinformatics tools for investigating the interaction of lncRNAs with other molecules.

The formation of RNA-dsDNA triplex is sequence-specific. Some motifs are easier to form triplex [77]. Therefore, the bioinformatics method can be used to predict the binding sites. Triplexator [78] and Longtarget [79] are two bioinformatics tools that have been used to predict lncRNA-dsDNA bindings. There are a number of bioinformatics tools to predict RNA-RNA interaction, such as RNAup [80], intaRNA [81], RNAplex [82], etc. RNAup calculates the thermodynamics of RNA-RNA interactions. IntaRNA is a fast approach for predicting RNA-RNA interaction incorporating accessibility and seeding of interaction sites. Recently, Gawronski et al. proposed a pipeline (MechRNA) to predict lncRNA interactions with target RNA using IntaRNA2, as well as the protein bindings with other tools [83]. The performance of various RNA-RNA interaction tools has been summarized previously [84].

Based on ceRNA hypothesis and seed region match rule, many databases and bioinformatics tools have been developed. Targetscan [68], starBase [85], miRTar-Base [86], Pictar [87], miRanda [88] and other bioinformatics tools have been used for the prediction of miRNA targets. Our group developed a novel network-based method previously to integrate the correlations between lncRNA, protein coding genes and miRNA [71]. We also designed a model to assess the combined impact of mRNAs, lncRNAs and miRNAs on cellular signaling transduction networks recently [71]. Tong et al. developed tools and a server to enable validating predicted lncRNA-miRNA-mRNA regulations from TCGA RNA-seq data and identifying miRNA-associated cancer signaling pathways and related lncRNA sponges [89, 90]. However, because of the complicate reticular networks, it is difficult to evaluate the effect of individual ceRNAs based solely on the bioinformatics analysis [91, 92].

Bioinformatics sciences have developed various tools for predicting ncRNA-protein interaction. Most of the existing methods are based on the sequences of either proteins or RNAs. Some of them investigate the associations between proteins and RNAs, such as RPI-Pred [93], RPIseq [94], and lncPro [95]. Some tools are used to predict binding sites of RNAs or proteins, such as BindN [96], RNABindR [97], RNAProB [98], PPRint [99], PRINTR [100], PRBR [101], SRCPred [102], RNABindRPlus [103] and RBRIdent [104]. The CatRAPID [105] method is specially designed to determine residue-nucleotide interactions. We developed a three-step prediction model called RPI-Bind for the identification of RNA-protein binding regions based on both sequences and structures of proteins and RNAs. These three steps include: (1) prediction of RNA binding regions on proteins, (2) prediction of protein binding regions on RNA, and (3) simultaneous prediction of interaction regions on RNA and proteins [106]. Suresh et al. developed a RNA-protein interaction predictor (RPI-Pred) using a new support-vector machine-based method to predict protein-RNA interaction pairs, based on both the sequences and structures [93]. The usage of machine learning algorithms have improved the prediction accuracies [93, 106].

7. Conclusions

Advances in high throughput technologies results in a rapid identification of a large amount of lncRNAs and expands our understanding of the mechanisms how lncRNAs function. Accumulating evidence indicates the complicated roles of lncRNAs. In order to gain deep insight into the interaction of lncRNA with other molecules, a number of bioinformatics tools have been developed. It is undeniable that our understanding of gene regulation by lncRNAs is still in the early stages. Given the growing numbers of lncRNA studies, we can anticipate that the detailed roles of novel lncRNAs will be addressed in the near future.

Acknowledgements

This work was partially supported by National Institutes of Health grants [NIH R01GM123037, U01AR069395-01A1, and U01CA166886] to X. Zhou.

Author details

Zhijin Li[1,2], Weiling Zhao[1], Maode Wang[2] and Xiaobo Zhou[1,3,4*]

1 Center for Computational Systems Medicine, School of Biomedical Informatics, The University of Texas Health Science Center at Houston, Houston, TX, USA

2 Department of Neurosurgery, The First Affiliated Hospital of Xi'an Jiaotong University, Xi'an, Shaanxi, China

3 McGovern Medical School, The University of Texas Health Science Center at Houston, Houston, TX, USA

4 School of Dentistry, The University of Texas Health Science Center at Houston, Houston, TX, USA

*Address all correspondence to: xiaobo.zhou@uth.tmc.edu

IntechOpen

© 2019 The Author(s). Licensee IntechOpen. This chapter is distributed under the terms of the Creative Commons Attribution License (http://creativecommons.org/licenses/by/3.0), which permits unrestricted use, distribution, and reproduction in any medium, provided the original work is properly cited. (cc) BY

References

[1] Green ED, Watson JD, Collins FS. Human genome project: Twenty-five years of big biology. Nature. 2015;**526**(7571):29-31

[2] Hangauer MJ, Vaughn IW, McManus MT. Pervasive transcription of the human genome produces thousands of previously unidentified long intergenic noncoding RNAs. PLoS Genetics. 2013;**9**(6):e1003569

[3] Mortazavi A et al. Mapping and quantifying mammalian transcriptomes by RNA-Seq. Nature Methods. 2008;**5**(7):621-628

[4] Djebali S et al. Landscape of transcription in human cells. Nature. 2012;**489**(7414):101-108

[5] Birney E et al. Identification and analysis of functional elements in 1% of the human genome by the ENCODE pilot project. Nature. 2007;**447**(7146):799-816

[6] Derrien T et al. The GENCODE v7 catalog of human long noncoding RNAs: Analysis of their gene structure, evolution, and expression. Genome Research. 2012;**22**(9):1775-1789

[7] Harrow J et al. GENCODE: The reference human genome annotation for the ENCODE project. Genome Research. 2012;**22**(9):1760-1774

[8] Volders PJ et al. An update on LNCipedia: A database for annotated human lncRNA sequences. Nucleic Acids Research. 2015;**43**(Database issue):D174-D180

[9] Volders PJ et al. LNCipedia: A database for annotated human lncRNA transcript sequences and structures. Nucleic Acids Research. 2013;**41**(Database issue):D246-D251

[10] Dianatpour A, Ghafouri-Fard S. The role of long non coding RNAs in the repair of DNA double strand breaks. International Journal of Molecular and Cellular Medicine. 2017;**6**(1):1-12

[11] Chen J, Liu S, Hu X. Long non-coding RNAs: Crucial regulators of gastrointestinal cancer cell proliferation. Cell Death Discovery. 2018;**4**:50

[12] Wang L et al. Missing links in epithelial-mesenchymal transition: Long non-coding RNAs enter the arena. Cellular Physiology and Biochemistry. 2017;**44**(4):1665-1680

[13] Xu T et al. Pathological bases and clinical impact of long noncoding RNAs in prostate cancer: A new budding star. Molecular Cancer. 2018;**17**(1):103

[14] Xie H et al. Long non-coding RNA CRNDE in cancer prognosis: Review and meta-analysis. Clinica Chimica Acta. 2018;**485**:262-271

[15] Huang H et al. Long noncoding RNAs and their epigenetic function in hematological diseases. 2018. DOI: 10.1002/hon.2534

[16] Archer K et al. Long non-coding RNAs as master regulators in cardiovascular diseases. International Journal of Molecular Sciences. 2015;**16**(10):23651-23667

[17] Beck D et al. A four-gene LincRNA expression signature predicts risk in multiple cohorts of acute myeloid leukemia patients. 2018;**32**(2):263-272

[18] Mou Y et al. Identification of long noncoding RNAs biomarkers in patients with hepatitis B virus-associated hepatocellular carcinoma. Cancer Biomarkers, 2018;**23**(1):95-106

[19] Jiang X, Lei R, Ning Q. Circulating long noncoding RNAs

as novel biomarkers of human diseases. Biomarkers in Medicine. 2016;**10**(7):757-769

[20] Wang KC, Chang HY. Molecular mechanisms of long noncoding RNAs. Molecular Cell. 2011;**43**(6):904-914

[21] Brockdorff N. Noncoding RNA and Polycomb recruitment. RNA. 2013;**19**(4):429-442

[22] Mercer TR, Mattick JS. Structure and function of long noncoding RNAs in epigenetic regulation. Nature Structural & Molecular Biology. 2013;**20**(3):300-307

[23] Ulitsky I, Bartel DP. lincRNAs: Genomics, evolution, and mechanisms. Cell. 2013;**154**(1):26-46

[24] Wang L et al. LncRNA Dum interacts with Dnmts to regulate Dppa2 expression during myogenic differentiation and muscle regeneration. Cell Research. 2015;**25**(3):335-350

[25] Tsai MC et al. Long noncoding RNA as modular scaffold of histone modification complexes. Science. 2010;**329**(5992):689-693

[26] Rinn JL et al. Functional demarcation of active and silent chromatin domains in human HOX loci by noncoding RNAs. Cell. 2007;**129**(7):1311-1323

[27] Wang KC et al. A long noncoding RNA maintains active chromatin to coordinate homeotic gene expression. Nature. 2011;**472**(7341):120-124

[28] Berghoff EG et al. Evf2 (Dlx6as) lncRNA regulates ultraconserved enhancer methylation and the differential transcriptional control of adjacent genes. Development. 2013;**140**(21):4407-4416

[29] Sun TT et al. LncRNA GClnc1 promotes gastric carcinogenesis and

may act as a modular scaffold of WDR5 and KAT2A complexes to specify the histone modification pattern. Cancer Discovery. 2016;**6**(7):784-801

[30] Zhao Z et al. lncRNA PAPAS tethered to the rDNA enhancer recruits hypophosphorylated CHD4/NuRD to repress rRNA synthesis at elevated temperatures. Genes & Development. 2018;**32**(11-12):836-848

[31] Zhou Y et al. Activation of p53 by MEG3 non-coding RNA. The Journal of Biological Chemistry. 2007;**282**(34):24731-24742

[32] Cabianca DS et al. A long ncRNA links copy number variation to a polycomb/trithorax epigenetic switch in FSHD muscular dystrophy. Cell. 2012;**149**(4):819-831

[33] Gong C et al. A long non-coding RNA, LncMyoD, regulates skeletal muscle differentiation by blocking IMP2-mediated mRNA translation. Developmental Cell. 2015;**34**(2):181-191

[34] Shih JW et al. Long noncoding RNA LncHIFCAR/MIR31HG is a HIF-1alpha co-activator driving oral cancer progression. Nature Communications. 2017;**8**:15874

[35] Miao Y et al. Enhancer-associated long non-coding RNA LEENE regulates endothelial nitric oxide synthase and endothelial function. 2018;**9**(1):292

[36] Cho SW et al. Promoter of lncRNA gene PVT1 is a tumor-suppressor DNA boundary element. Cell. 2018;**173**(6):1398-1412.e22

[37] Tripathi V et al. Long noncoding RNA MALAT1 controls cell cycle progression by regulating the expression of oncogenic transcription factor B-MYB. PLoS Genetics. 2013;**9**(3):e1003368

[38] Ciarlo E et al. An intronic ncRNA-dependent regulation of SORL1 expression affecting Abeta formation is upregulated in post-mortem Alzheimer's disease brain samples. Disease Models & Mechanisms. 2013;**6**(2):424-433

[39] Cao L et al. LAST, a c-Myc-inducible long noncoding RNA, cooperates with CNBP to promote CCND1 mRNA stability in human cells. eLife. 2017;**6**:e30433

[40] Faghihi MA et al. Evidence for natural antisense transcript-mediated inhibition of microRNA function. Genome Biology. 2010;**11**(5):R56

[41] Faghihi MA et al. Expression of a noncoding RNA is elevated in Alzheimer's disease and drives rapid feed-forward regulation of beta-secretase. Nature Medicine. 2008;**14**(7):723-730

[42] Matsui K et al. Natural antisense transcript stabilizes inducible nitric oxide synthase messenger RNA in rat hepatocytes. Hepatology. 2008;**47**(2):686-697

[43] Rossignol F, Vache C, Clottes E. Natural antisense transcripts of hypoxia-inducible factor 1alpha are detected in different normal and tumour human tissues. Gene. 2002;**299**(1-2):135-140

[44] Zhang A et al. LncRNA HOTAIR enhances the androgen-receptor-mediated transcriptional program and drives castration-resistant prostate cancer. Cell Reports. 2015;**13**(1):209-221

[45] Liu L et al. LncRNA MT1JP functions as a tumor suppressor by interacting with TIAR to modulate the p53 pathway. Oncotarget. 2016;**7**(13):15787-15800

[46] Yang F et al. Reciprocal regulation of HIF-1alpha and lincRNA-p21 modulates the Warburg effect. Molecular Cell. 2014;**53**(1):88-100

[47] Li D et al. Activity dependent LoNA regulates translation by coordinating rRNA transcription and methylation. Nature Communications. 2018;**9**(1):1726

[48] Tran NT et al. The AS-RBM15 lncRNA enhances RBM15 protein translation during megakaryocyte differentiation. 2016;**17**(6):887-900

[49] Carrieri C et al. Long non-coding antisense RNA controls Uchl1 translation through an embedded SINEB2 repeat. Nature. 2012;**491**(7424):454-457

[50] Hu G, Lou Z, Gupta M. The long non-coding RNA GAS5 cooperates with the eukaryotic translation initiation factor 4E to regulate c-Myc translation. PLoS One. 2014;**9**(9):e107016

[51] Yamamura S et al. Interaction and cross-talk between non-coding RNAs. Cellular and Molecular Life Sciences. 2018;**75**(3):467-484

[52] Zhou W et al. The lncRNA H19 mediates breast cancer cell plasticity during EMT and MET plasticity by differentially sponging miR-200b/c and let-7b. 2017;**10**(483). DOI: 10.1126/scisignal.aak9557

[53] Ma C et al. H19 promotes pancreatic cancer metastasis by derepressing let-7's suppression on its target HMGA2-mediated EMT. Tumour Biology. 2014;**35**(9):9163-9169

[54] Morriss GR, Cooper TA. Protein sequestration as a normal function of long noncoding RNAs and a pathogenic mechanism of RNAs containing nucleotide repeat expansions. Human Genetics. 2017;**136**(9):1247-1263

[55] Lee S et al. Noncoding RNA NORAD regulates genomic stability by

sequestering PUMILIO proteins. Cell. 2016;**164**(1-2):69-80

[56] Zhou J et al. H19 lncRNA alters DNA methylation genome wide by regulating S-adenosylhomocysteine hydrolase. 2015;**6**:10221

[57] Kino T et al. Noncoding RNA gas5 is a growth arrest- and starvation-associated repressor of the glucocorticoid receptor. Science Signaling. 2010;**3**(107):ra8

[58] Duca M et al. The triple helix: 50 years later, the outcome. Nucleic Acids Research. 2008;**36**(16):5123-5138

[59] Roberts RW, Crothers DM. Stability and properties of double and triple helices: Dramatic effects of RNA or DNA backbone composition. Science. 1992;**258**(5087):1463-1466

[60] Martianov I et al. Repression of the human dihydrofolate reductase gene by a non-coding interfering transcript. Nature. 2007;**445**(7128):666-670

[61] Grote P, Herrmann BG. The long non-coding RNA Fendrr links epigenetic control mechanisms to gene regulatory networks in mammalian embryogenesis. RNA Biology. 2013;**10**(10):1579-1585

[62] Grote P et al. The tissue-specific lncRNA Fendrr is an essential regulator of heart and body wall development in the mouse. Developmental Cell. 2013;**24**(2):206-214

[63] Simon MD et al. The genomic binding sites of a noncoding RNA. Proceedings of the National Academy of Sciences of the United States of America. 2011;**108**(51):20497-20502

[64] Salmena L et al. A ceRNA hypothesis: The Rosetta stone of a hidden RNA language? Cell. 2011;**146**(3):353-358

[65] Filipowicz W, Bhattacharyya SN, Sonenberg N. Mechanisms of post-transcriptional regulation by microRNAs: Are the answers in sight? Nature Reviews. Genetics. 2008;**9**(2):102-114

[66] Ahadi A, Sablok G, Hutvagner G. miRTar2GO: A novel rule-based model learning method for cell line specific microRNA target prediction that integrates Ago2 CLIP-Seq and validated microRNA-target interaction data. Nucleic Acids Research. 2017;**45**(6):e42

[67] Zhang XQ, Yang JH. Discovering circRNA-microRNA interactions from CLIP-Seq data. Methods in Molecular Biology. 2018;**1724**:193-207

[68] Lewis BP, Burge CB, Bartel DP. Conserved seed pairing, often flanked by adenosines, indicates that thousands of human genes are microRNA targets. Cell. 2005;**120**(1):15-20

[69] Beltran M et al. A natural antisense transcript regulates Zeb2/Sip1 gene expression during Snail1-induced epithelial-mesenchymal transition. Genes & Development. 2008;**22**(6):756-769

[70] Gong C, Maquat LE. lncRNAs transactivate STAU1-mediated mRNA decay by duplexing with 3' UTRs via Alu elements. Nature. 2011;**470**(7333):284-288

[71] Sharma E et al. Global mapping of human RNA-RNA interactions. Molecular Cell. 2016;**62**(4):618-626

[72] Nguyen TC et al. Mapping RNA-RNA interactome and RNA structure in vivo by MARIO. Nature Communications. 2016;**7**:12023

[73] Wang C et al. LncRNA structural characteristics in epigenetic regulation. International Journal of Molecular Sciences. 2017;**18**(12). DOI: 10.3390/ijms18122659

[74] Ferre F, Colantoni A, Helmer-Citterich M. Revealing protein-lncRNA interaction. Briefings in Bioinformatics. 2016;**17**(1):106-116

[75] Zhang T, Tan P, Wang L. RNALocate: A resource for RNA subcellular localizations. 2017;**45**(D1):D135-d138

[76] Su ZD et al. iLoc-lncRNA: Predict the subcellular location of lncRNAs by incorporating octamer composition into general PseKNC. Bioinformatics. 2018. DOI: 10.1093/bioinformatics/bty508

[77] Li Y, Syed J, Sugiyama H. RNA-DNA triplex formation by long noncoding RNAs. Cell Chemical Biology. 2016;**23**(11):1325-1333

[78] Buske FA et al. Triplexator: Detecting nucleic acid triple helices in genomic and transcriptomic data. Genome Research. 2012;**22**(7):1372-1381

[79] He S et al. LongTarget: A tool to predict lncRNA DNA-binding motifs and binding sites via Hoogsteen base-pairing analysis. Bioinformatics. 2015;**31**(2):178-186

[80] Muckstein U et al. Thermodynamics of RNA-RNA binding. Bioinformatics. 2006;**22**(10):1177-1182

[81] Busch A, Richter AS, Backofen R. IntaRNA: Efficient prediction of bacterial sRNA targets incorporating target site accessibility and seed regions. Bioinformatics. 2008;**24**(24):2849-2856

[82] Tafer H, Hofacker IL. RNAplex: A fast tool for RNA-RNA interaction search. Bioinformatics. 2008;**24**(22):2657-2663

[83] Gawronski AR et al. MechRNA: Prediction of lncRNA mechanisms from RNA-RNA and RNA-protein interactions. Bioinformatics, 2018; **34**(18):3101-3110

[84] Umu SU, Gardner PP. A comprehensive benchmark of RNA-RNA interaction prediction tools for all domains of life. Bioinformatics. 2017;**33**(7):988-996

[85] Li JH et al. starBase v2.0: Decoding miRNA-ceRNA, miRNA-ncRNA and protein-RNA interaction networks from large-scale CLIP-Seq data. Nucleic Acids Research. 2014;**42**(Database issue):D92-D97

[86] Hsu SD et al. miRTarBase: A database curates experimentally validated microRNA-target interactions. Nucleic Acids Research. 2011;**39**(Database issue):D163-D169

[87] Krek A et al. Combinatorial microRNA target predictions. Nature Genetics. 2005;**37**(5):495-500

[88] John B et al. Human microRNA targets. PLoS Biology. 2004;**2**(11):e363

[89] Liu K et al. Annotating function to differentially expressed LincRNAs in myelodysplastic syndrome using a network-based method. Bioinformatics. 2017;**33**(17):2622-2630

[90] Tong Y, Ru B, Zhang J. miRNACancerMAP: an integrative web server inferring miRNA regulation network for cancer. Bioinformatics, 2018;**34**(18):3211-3213

[91] Tay Y, Rinn J, Pandolfi PP. The multilayered complexity of ceRNA crosstalk and competition. Nature. 2014;**505**(7483):344-352

[92] Thomson DW, Dinger ME. Endogenous microRNA sponges: Evidence and controversy. Nature Reviews. Genetics. 2016;**17**(5):272-283

[93] Suresh V et al. RPI-Pred: Predicting ncRNA-protein interaction using sequence and structural information. Nucleic Acids Research. 2015;**43**(3):1370-1379

[94] Livi CM, Blanzieri E. Protein-specific prediction of mRNA binding using RNA sequences, binding motifs and predicted secondary structures. BMC Bioinformatics. 2014;**15**:123

[95] Lu Q et al. Computational prediction of associations between long non-coding RNAs and proteins. BMC Genomics. 2013;**14**:651

[96] Wang L, Brown SJ. BindN: A web-based tool for efficient prediction of DNA and RNA binding sites in amino acid sequences. Nucleic Acids Research. 2006;**34**(Web Server issue):W243-W248

[97] Terribilini M et al. RNABindR: A server for analyzing and predicting RNA-binding sites in proteins. Nucleic Acids Research. 2007;**35**(Web Server issue):W578-W584

[98] Liu ZP et al. Prediction of protein-RNA binding sites by a random forest method with combined features. Bioinformatics. 2010;**26**(13):1616-1622

[99] Kumar M, Gromiha MM, Raghava GP. Prediction of RNA binding sites in a protein using SVM and PSSM profile. Proteins. 2008;**71**(1):189-194

[100] Wang Y et al. PRINTR: Prediction of RNA binding sites in proteins using SVM and profiles. Amino Acids. 2008;**35**(2):295-302

[101] Ma X et al. Prediction of RNA-binding residues in proteins from primary sequence using an enriched random forest model with a novel hybrid feature. Proteins. 2011;**79**(4):1230-1239

[102] Fernandez M et al. Prediction of dinucleotide-specific RNA-binding sites in proteins. BMC Bioinformatics. 2011;**12**(Suppl. 13):S5

[103] Walia RR et al. RNABindRPlus: A predictor that combines machine learning and sequence homology-based methods to improve the reliability of predicted RNA-binding residues in proteins. PLoS One. 2014;**9**(5):e97725

[104] Xiong D, Zeng J, Gong H. RBRIdent: An algorithm for improved identification of RNA-binding residues in proteins from primary sequences. Proteins. 2015;**83**(6):1068-1077

[105] Livi CM et al. catRAPID signature: Identification of ribonucleoproteins and RNA-binding regions. Bioinformatics. 2016;**32**(5):773-775

[106] Luo J et al. RPI-bind: A structure-based method for accurate identification of RNA-protein binding sites. Scientific Reports. 2017;**7**(1):614

Section 3

Genes and Cancer

Chapter 4

Genes That Can Cause Cancer

Chanda Siddoo-Atwal

Abstract

Recently, it has become apparent that the pathogenesis of cancer is closely connected with aberrantly regulated apoptotic cell death and the resulting deregulation of cell proliferation. The loss of equilibrium between cell proliferation and cell death in a tissue may play a crucial role in tumor formation. In fact, the initiation of uncontrolled apoptosis in a tissue may serve as the trigger for carcinogenesis. Various laboratory studies on animals and certain human data are suggestive that tumor formation requires at least two discrete events to take place in response to a carcinogen according to this apoptotic model of carcinogenesis. The first involves an elevation of apoptosis in a particular tissue due to a genetic predisposition, stress, or mutation. The second confers resistance to apoptosis in that same tissue resulting in the formation of an abnormal growth due to a dysregulation of cell number homeostasis. The apoptotic response of each individual to any given carcinogenic or other environmental stimulus is determined by their unique double set of genes inherited from both parents. The singular genetic traits and biochemistry of each individual are attributable solely to this unique combination of genes and their specific regulation. A general example of genetic regulation, gene dose, and control is provided by β-thalassemia point mutations in the beta-globin gene, which confer a blood disease mainly in Mediterranean populations. This mutation (heterozygous and homozygous, at one or both genetic loci) can cause a hereditary red blood cell anemia. Specific examples in relation to cancer predisposition include various genetic models such as the elevated levels of skin cancer among those with certain polymorphisms or inherited mutations in their DNA repair genes like those associated with the disorder, Xeroderma pigmentosum (XP); the high rate of skin cancer observed in albinos with little or no melanin; and the high incidence of lymphomas occurring in patients with the inherited disorder, ataxia-telangiectasia (AT). The mutations associated with each of these conditions can result in an elevated level of apoptosis in the target tissues, either constitutively or in response to particular carcinogens such as UV rays, and can be linked to the initiation of cancer in those specific tissues.

Keywords: apoptosis, carcinogenesis, albinism, β-thalassemia, Xeroderma pigmentosum, trichothiodystrophy, DNA repair polymorphisms, DNA repair defect ataxia-telangiectasia

1. Current models of carcinogenesis

Classically, experimental carcinogenesis is a complex, multistage process including initiation, promotion, and malignant progression in which the failure of DNA repair mechanisms and the subsequent clonal expansion of damaged cells play a pivotal role. However, more recently, it has become apparent that the pathogenesis

IntechOpen

of cancer is closely connected with aberrantly regulated apoptotic cell death and the resulting deregulation of cell proliferation [1, 2].

The Ames assay as a universal test for carcinogenicity was based on the classical model of carcinogenesis involving the failure of DNA repair mechanisms and the subsequent clonal expansion of mutated cells. However, mutagenicity in bacterial strains is not always an indicator of carcinogenicity since many carcinogens are not mutagenic [5]. Although this may be one feasible mechanism of carcinogenesis in laboratory models, it does not adequately fit many existing systems of carcinogenesis which are increasingly connected with aberrantly regulated apoptotic cell death and the resulting deregulation of cell proliferation. Evidence for the role of apoptotic dysregulation in carcinogenesis comes from several sources involving epidemiological, histological, and comparative animal studies in different target organs. A number of human and mouse models also support a correlation between an initial elevation in apoptosis and subsequent tumorigenesis in various tissues as in the case of the human skin cancer model [6].

Logically, in the initial stages of carcinogenesis, the most important factor to consider may be that of "time." Gene-specific mutations are known to occur randomly over a long period of time, sometimes spanning several generations according to Darwinian doctrine. There simply may not be enough time even over the life-span of a single organism to produce a specific mutation, and it seems less likely that a specific mutation to initiate carcinogenesis could happen in response to a particular carcinogen. Even according to Lamarck's alternate theory of "acquired characteristics" in which altered genetic characteristics acquired over a length of time by a parent may be passed on to the next generation, it is a stretch at best. However, if following exposure to a carcinogen, which causes the generation of free radicals and DNA damage, the occurrence of a specific mutation becomes more likely; this likelihood is still greater at a later point in time. In effect, a specific mutation would be more likely to occur at a later stage of carcinogenesis than during an earlier one. According to the two-stage model of tumor formation (see **Diagram 2**), while an epigenetic change is more likely to occur in the first step of carcinogenesis, a genetic mutation is more likely to occur in the second step of carcinogenesis merely as a function of probability [7].

2. An apoptotic model of carcinogenesis

"Apoptosis" (*falling leaves* in Greek) specifically refers to one particular mode of cell death which is responsible for the elimination of potentially deleterious, mutated cells in multicellular organisms. Inducers of apoptosis include intracellular and extracellular stimuli such as DNA damage, oxidative stress, cell cycle disruption, hypoxia, detachment from surrounding tissue, and loss of trophic signaling [8]. Apoptosis is regulated through at least two well-recognized pathways, both involving caspase activation. The first of these is called the "intrinsic pathway" and is mediated through mitochondrial release of cytochrome c, while the second is known as the "extrinsic pathway" and is mediated through cell surface death receptors, such as the receptor for tumor necrosis factor (TNF) [9, 10]. More recently, a caspase-independent apoptotic pathway has also been gaining some prominence in apoptosis studies [11].

Apoptosis is involved in the homeostasis of cell number in tissues, and although, increased cell proliferation is necessary, it is certainly not sufficient for cell transformation to take place. Normally, in multicellular organisms, a dynamic equilibrium exists between cell birth and cell death to maintain constant cell numbers throughout adult life. This homeostasis depends on an integrated balance between

A.   B.   C.   D.

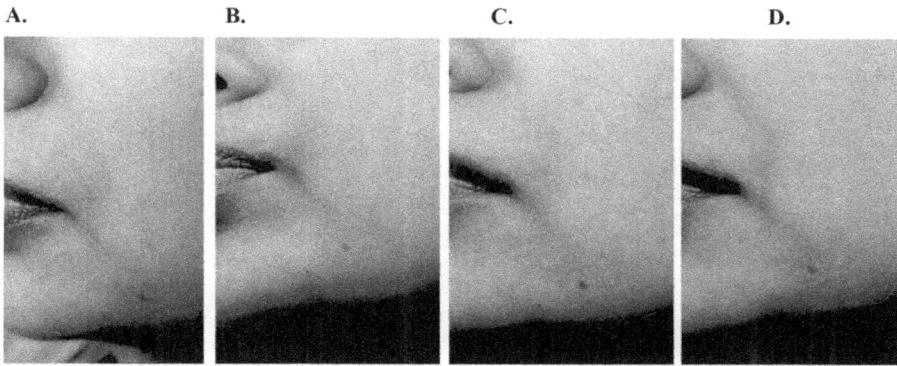

Figure 1.
The human sunburn cycle. (A) 48 h, redness & inflammation; (B) 96 h, new tissue formation; apoptosis (onset); (C) 120 h, apoptosis; (D) 168 h, apoptosis (end). The natural human sunburn cycle (without the use of any sun lotions or sunscreens) is approximately 1 week in length (7 days) from start to finish. Macroscopically, it consists of three phases including Inflammation, New Tissue Formation, and Apoptosis (visible peeling). The inflammatory phase consists of redness and inflammation commencing 20–30 minutes from the time of initial sun exposure. It spans grossly 2–3 days but can last up to 5 or 6 days depending upon UV intensity. New tissue formation is stimulated some time after initial exposure, and it is complete within 1 week. In the last apoptotic phase, the top layer of dead skin cells sloughs off to reveal a new tissue layer beneath. This process follows on from the inflammatory phase and is complete approximately 7 days following sun exposure. (The photos below are based on an initial exposure time of 20–30 min at a Canadian beach in February.)

apoptosis and mitosis such that these two activities are counterbalanced and equivalent. This homeostatic balance may contribute a critical defense mechanism of the cell to various genotoxic agents such as carcinogens [3].

The increased proliferation in some preneoplastic lesions is often accompanied by a parallel increase in apoptosis. A permanent loss in homeostatic equilibrium between cell proliferation and death may be a critical determinant in the transition to tumorigenesis. Support for this comes from the islet B cells of a multistage mouse model of carcinogenesis in which the incidence of apoptosis increased in parallel with increasing proliferation during tumor promotion, while malignancy was associated with a dramatic drop in apoptotic rate without a corresponding decrease in proliferation rate [4]. Also, in the natural human skin cancer model (*not* involving the application of inflammatory skin irritants or tumor promoters found in various suntan oils), there is always a fresh layer of new epidermis underlying the peeling or apoptosing cells as part of the normal human sunburn cycle in response to sunlight (see **Figure 1** and **Diagram 1**) [12]. Tumor formation only seems to occur once the cancer cells display constitutively activated apoptosis and become resistant to apoptosis while continuing to proliferate. In fact, acquired resistance to apoptosis appears to be a pivotal event in immortalization and the transition to malignancy [3, 13].

Various laboratory studies on animals and certain human data are suggestive that tumor formation requires at least two discrete events to take place in response to a carcinogen according to the apoptotic model of carcinogenesis. The first involves an elevation of apoptosis in a particular tissue due to a genetic predisposition, stress, or mutation in response to a carcinogen. The second confers resistance to apoptosis in that same tissue resulting in the formation of an abnormal growth due to a dysregulation of cell number homeostasis (see **Diagram 2**). Moreover, there is some evidence to suggest that both these events can be reversible when treated with a selective apoptotic agent (see **Diagram 3**), and, hence, they may be either genetic or epigenetic in nature [6].

In this context, uncontrolled apoptosis has been directly linked to carcinogenesis. Scientific animal studies have shown that simply increasing the basal frequency

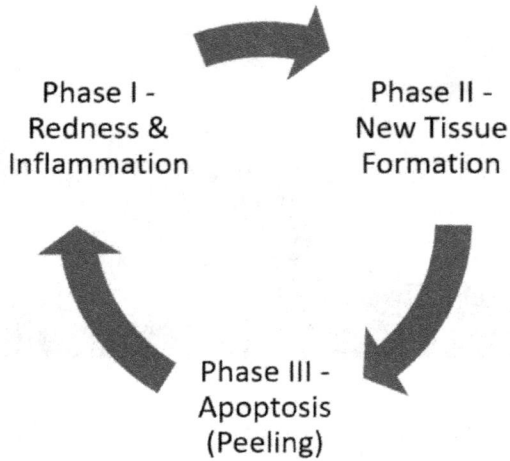

Phase I -
Redness &
Inflammation

Phase II -
New Tissue
Formation

Phase III -
Apoptosis
(Peeling)

Diagram 1.
The human sunburn cycle. If this cycle continues unchecked in a specific exposed area on the body, it may result in skin cancer.

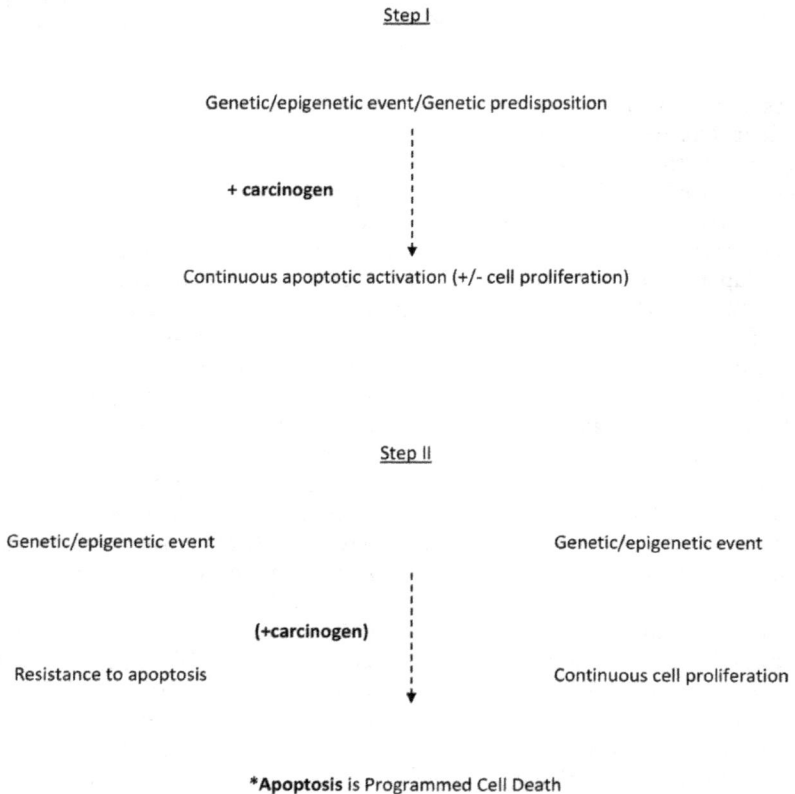

Step I

Genetic/epigenetic event/Genetic predisposition

+ carcinogen

Continuous apoptotic activation (+/- cell proliferation)

Step II

Genetic/epigenetic event

Genetic/epigenetic event

(+carcinogen)

Resistance to apoptosis

Continuous cell proliferation

*Apoptosis is Programmed Cell Death

Diagram 2.
Two-stage model of tumor formation (expanded version). Apoptosis is programmed cell death.

of apoptosis in murine skin cells can be linked to the development of squamous cell carcinomas in transgenic mice [14]. In fact, the proliferation rate in certain tissues like nerve cells is so slow or negligible that simply an elevation of apoptosis would

<u>Step I</u>

Genetic/epigenetic event/Genetic predisposition

Selective Apoptotic

Agent

Continuous apoptotic activation

<u>Step II</u>

Genetic/epigenetic event

Selective

Apoptotic

Agent

Resistance to apoptosis

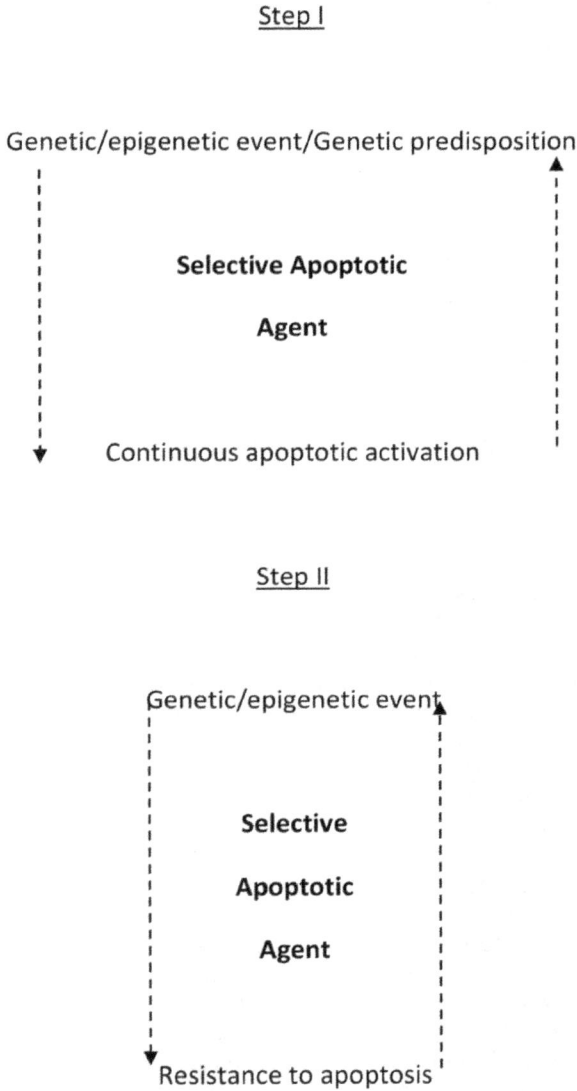

Diagram 3.
Two-stage model of tumor formation and action of selective apoptotic agent.

be sufficient to disrupt the balance between cell birth and death in the brain or nervous system even prior to the second step in the two-stage model of carcinogenesis connected with resistance to apoptosis and tumor formation.

Thus, according to this new model, the stimulation of apoptotic mechanisms becomes an important focus of study and key determinant of carcinogenic potential for any particular carcinogen being studied [15].

3. An example of gene regulation

The apoptotic response of each individual to any given carcinogenic or other environmental stimulus is determined by their unique double set of genes inherited from their parents. The singular genetic traits and biochemistry of each individual are attributable solely to this unique combination of genes and their specific regulation. A general example of genetic regulation, gene dose, and control is provided by β-thalassemia mutations in the beta-globin gene, which confer a blood disease mainly in Mediterranean populations.

4. β-Thalassemia

Beta-thalassemias are a group of hereditary blood disorders affecting the synthesis of beta hemoglobin chains, and the results range from severe anemias requiring regular blood transfusions to asymptomatic individuals [16]. There are three main forms of the disease: thalassemia major, the most severe form with early presentation; thalassemia intermedia, a moderate form with clinical symptoms that present later in life; and, thalassemia minor, the least severe and asymptomatic form, which can cause moderate anemia. Frequency of this disease is 1 in 10,000 in the European Union and 1 in 100,000 throughout the rest of the world. Beta-thalassemias are caused mainly by point mutations and more rarely by deletions in the beta-globin gene on chromosome 11 leading to reduced or absent synthesis of beta hemoglobin chains. The transmission of this genetic trait is usually autosomal recessive, but dominant mutations also exist.

In developing countries where diagnosis of thalassemia major can be delayed, clinically, children may display growth retardation, pallor, jaundice, poor musculature, leg ulcers, and skeletal changes among other symptoms. In developed countries where blood transfusions may be implemented sooner, patients can develop iron overload-related issues including endocrine complications, dilated myocardiopathy, liver fibrosis, and cirrhosis. The main clinical features of thalassemia intermedia patients are hypertrophy of erythroid marrow and related complications, gallstones, painful leg ulcers, and an increased predisposition to thrombosis. Thalassemia minor is not associated with any clinical symptoms except mild or moderate anemia in certain cases.

The a- and b-globin genes are expressed exclusively in erythroid cells and only during defined periods of development to ensure the correct balance of a- and b-globin chains which form the tetramer of various hemoglobins at different stages. Such tight control of these multigene clusters requires several levels of regulation [17]. This is dependent on regulatory regions of DNA lying in proximity or at great distances from the globin genes. The latter are characterized by several DNase I hypersensitive sites and form the locus control region (LCR). The former and latter sequences exert stimulatory, inhibitory, or more complex activities by interacting with transcription factors that bridge these DNA regions to the RNA polymerase machinery of the cell. Also, LCR can make physical contact with active downstream globin genes by forming a chromatin structure called the active chromatin hub (ACH) in a process termed chromatin looping [18].

The coding sequences of globin genes are generally found within three exons, separated by two introns. Each gene has 5′ promoter sequences, 5′ and 3′ untranslated regions, and a downstream enhancer, in the case of the b-globin gene, which is approximately 600–900 base pairs 3′ of the poly(A) site [19].

GATA transcription factors bind the consensus sequence WGATAR, which is present in the flanking regions of most erythroid-specific genes. Conserved GATA sites are located in each of the hypersensitive sites of both alpha- and beta-globin gene clusters. GATA-1 and GATA-2 transcription factors are coexpressed in erythroid cells and are important for the regulation of erythroid globin genes, in particular for the modulation of embryonic and fetal hemoglobins [20].

β-Thalassemia is mainly caused by non-deletional defects of the b-globin gene, mostly single base substitutions. More than 180 mutations have been identified and classified as beta + or beta 0 depending on whether they reduce or abolish b-globin chain production, respectively. These mutants can be categorized as (1) nonsense or frameshift mutations which produce premature terminations, (2) RNA processing mutants which disrupt splicing and interfere with RNA cleavage or polyadenylation, (3) transcriptional mutants which disrupt the function of the promoter, and (4) mutations in the initiation codon or Cap site [21].

For example, thalassemia intermedia (homozygous and heterozygous forms) can be caused by mutations in the promoter region (CACCC or TATA box) of the beta-globin gene and have been reported in a Spanish population [19]. Nuclear proteins related to SP1 and GT-1 factors bind to a CACCC box sequence in the human beta-globin enhancer adjacent to the erythroid-specific factor NFE-1 and ubiquitous CP1. These same proteins bind to the proximal, but not distal, CACCC box in the human beta-globin promoter. A CG mutation in the promoter CACCC box known to cause beta-thalassemia greatly decreases protein binding. Similarly, the same effect is produced when this mutation is introduced into the enhancer CACCC box [22].

A study in Germany with nonimmigrant German populations found that roughly two-thirds of thalassemia minor cases appear to be caused by Mediterranean mutations (61%), while approximately a third of cases may have originated as a result of local mutations such as the one that affects position −2 of the intron 1 splice acceptor site (IVSI-129 A-G) and a deletion of a single G in codon 15/16 (FS 15/16 ΔG). The former finding suggests introduction due to migration from the Mediterranean region [23]. Similarly, while common mutations causing β-thalassemia major and minor occur in populations from northern, western, and eastern India, rare and even novel mutations may occur in some of these populations. In one Indian study, DNA sequencing of LCR HS2, 3, and 4 core sequences revealed a polymorphism, an A-G, in the palindromic sequence, TGGGGACCCCA, of LCR HS4 [24]. So, once again, the G allele could be a new evolutionary mutation in the Indian population, while the other mutations may have been introduced via migration, for example, as a result of intermarriages documented to have occurred in the frontier provinces during the Indo-Greek and Scythian periods of Indian history [25–27].

Thus, the multiple levels of gene regulation as illustrated in this example of the b-globin genes make up a highly and finely tuned system to determine subtle differences in gene expression between individuals resulting in varied production of b-globin chains. Such small differences or genetic polymorphisms are the reason for the genetic susceptibility of certain individuals to specific diseases. Similarly, in the human skin cancer model, the melanin pigment is the natural sunscreen of the human body, and the body protects itself from solar radiation by increasing melanin production. The UV A and UV B components of sunlight can trigger the human sunburn cycle involving three phases including cell death or apoptosis, repeatedly, in susceptible individuals (see **Table 1**), and this can result in skin cancer. Melanin ranges in color from red and yellow (pheomelanin) to brown and black (eumelanin) with the latter being the most effective [28]. However, certain individuals have less melanin than others and are not able to produce enough melanin to fulfill this function resulting in sunburn. In fact, it is possible and worth noting that certain forms of medical conditions such as actinic prurigo and cheilitis prevalent among some Native American populations [29] may actually be misdiagnosed cases of human sunburn. Notably, the pinkish or reddish hue of Native Americans (originally called "Red Indians" by the paler European settlers), a heightened degree of photosensitivity, and regular peeling of the epidermis upon exposure to sunlight all suggest a

0–1 h (Initial exposure)	Redness and inflammation
24 h (Day 1)	Redness and inflammation; pain
48 h (Day 2)	Redness and inflammation peak; pain
72 h (Day 3)	Minor peeling; less redness and inflammation
96 h (Day 4)	Major peeling
120 h (Day 5)	Minor peeling; itching
140 h (Day 6)	Minor peeling; itching
168 h (Day 7)	Recovery; visible new tissue

No use of sun preparations, sunscreen, or suntan lotion.
Approximately a 1-week/7-day cycle without the use of any sun preparations.

Table 1.
The human sunburn cycle.

I	Inflammation	0–72 h
II	New tissue formation	24–168 h
III	Apoptosis	36–168 h

This table is based on an initial exposure of 20–30 min at noon at the beach.
[These data are based on a set of experiments conducted at Ambleside Beach in West Vancouver (British Columbia), Canada, in February 2010.]

Table 2.
The three phases of sunburn.

lack of melanin in their skins. Since an elevation of apoptotic levels in mammalian skin cells has been linked to carcinogenesis, such patients predisposed to peeling require "apoptosis protection factor" (also called "tumor protection factor," previously) in their sunscreens as opposed to "sun protection factor," which mainly provides protection against redness and inflammation. Unfortunately, skin cancer statistics are not widely available for any Native American populations of North America at present (**Table 2**).

5. Examples of genes that can control apoptosis

Specific examples in relation to cancer predisposition include various genetic models such as the elevated levels of skin cancer among those with certain polymorphisms or inherited mutations in their DNA repair genes like those associated with the disorder, Xeroderma pigmentosum (XP); the high rate of skin cancer observed in albinos with little or no melanin; and the high incidence of lymphomas occurring in patients with the inherited disorder, ataxia-telangiectasia (AT). The mutations associated with each of these conditions can result in an elevated level of apoptosis in the target tissues, either constitutively or in response to particular carcinogens such as UV rays, and can be linked to the initiation of cancer in those specific tissues.

6. DNA repair defects and DNA repair polymorphisms

Mutations in the XPD helicase component of the transcription factor TFIIH, which is involved in basal transcription and DNA repair, can result in the diverse symptoms associated with both Xeroderma pigmentosum (XP) and trichothiodystrophy (TTD). Aside from the traditional mutations and deletions in the b-globin gene that induce β-thalassemia, it is interesting that specific mutations in XPD that cause TTD can also result in reduced expression of the b-globin gene, in addition to a number of other general clinical features. TTD is an autosomal recessive disorder characterized by brittle nails, brittle hair, short stature, mental retardation, ichthyotic skin, and, often, photosensitivity [30]. Photosensitive TTD patients tend to be deficient in nucleotide excision repair (NER) of UV-induced DNA damage and, in this aspect, resemble XP patients. XP is also an autosomal recessive disease that provides a useful cancer model and is characterized by extreme sensitivity of the skin to sunlight resulting in sunburn, sunlight-induced pigmentation changes in the skin, and a very high frequency of skin cancers in sun-exposed areas including basal or squamous cell carcinomas and melanomas. However, TTD patients display neither pigmentation changes nor skin cancers [31]. The explanation for this difference appears to lie in the fact that XPD has two functions and XP may be caused by mutations that only affect its role in NER, whereas TTD may be caused by mutations that affect its general transcriptional role as a subunit of the transcription factor TFIIH. In TTD patients, de novo synthesis of the components of TFIIH is thought to compensate for this deficiency in most cells, so there is little evidence for deficient transcription of many genes in TTD except for b-globin in humans [30]. Reduced repair of cyclobutane pyrimidine dimers (CPD), which do not seem to be cytotoxic on their own, is observed in TTD as well [32, 33]. By contrast, in XPA cells, entirely deficient in the repair of the two major UV-induced lesions, CPDs and (6–4) photoproducts, UV exposure results in cell death [34]. Moreover, 65% of the melanomas in patients with Xeroderma pigmentosum occur on areas that are routinely exposed to the sun like the face, head, or neck [35].

Epidemiological studies have also shown that homozygous genetic polymorphisms in DNA repair proteins resulting in sunburn, and a history of repeated painful sunburn are more correlated with a higher risk for squamous cell carcinoma than the wild-type or heterozygotes [36, 37]. In addition, variants within other DNA repair genes involved in double-stranded DNA repair triggered by UV damage have been found to be associated with the development of malignant melanoma [38]. Moreover, many cancers ranging from acute myeloid leukemia and follicular lymphoma to breast cancer have been associated with specific polymorphisms in DNA repair enzymes resulting in their reduced efficiency to cope with cellular DNA damage [39–41]. The inability to cope efficiently with DNA damage often results in cell death or apoptosis.

7. Albinism

There are a number of genetic models for skin cancer in humans. One such model is also provided by albinos, who are deficient in melanin production (melanin is the pigment that protects against UV radiation and apoptotic sunburn). Albinos are typically characterized by pink skin, pink eyes, and white hair resulting from mutations in genes involved in melanin biosynthesis [42]. As a result, they display an increased skin cancer incidence [43]. This finding is confirmed in the albino hairless mouse model which displays a high incidence of UV-induced cutaneous cancers as well [44].

8. Ataxia-telangiectasia

Patients with the inherited disorder ataxia-telangiectasia [AT] provide another human cancer model since they are highly susceptible to certain cancers, particularly lymphomas [45]. AT is an autosomal recessive disease which is characterized by loss of coordination and telangiectasias, hypersensitivity to ionizing radiation, progressive neuronal degeneration, and immunodeficiency [46]. Interestingly, the genetic mutation in AT patients occurs in and affects a PI 3-kinase associated with DNA damage and has been found to be involved in the apoptotic response to X-irradiation [47, 48].

In addition, a constitutive elevation of IFNβ production has been demonstrated in fibroblasts derived from AT individuals [49]. An elevation of spontaneous apoptosis in AT lymphocytes has also been observed [50] thereby establishing a link between apoptotic potential and an increase in cancer risk. Cytokines like IFNα/β are known to stimulate the transcription of many proapoptotic proteins [51]. The transcriptional activator, NF-κB, which mediates interferon (IFN) production, is constitutively activated in AT cells [52] as well and is apoptotic in certain cell types like lymphocytes [53]. Thus, there is further evidence here to suggest that cancer predisposition may be connected with genetic polymorphisms that can cause uncontrolled apoptosis.

Author details

Chanda Siddoo-Atwal
Moondust Cosmetics Ltd., Canada

*Address all correspondence to: moondustcosmetics@gmail.com

IntechOpen

© 2019 The Author(s). Licensee IntechOpen. This chapter is distributed under the terms of the Creative Commons Attribution License (http://creativecommons.org/licenses/by/3.0), which permits unrestricted use, distribution, and reproduction in any medium, provided the original work is properly cited. (cc) BY

References

[1] Denmeade SR, Isaacs JT. Programmed cell death (apoptosis) and cancer chemotherapy. Cancer Control. 1996;**3**(4):303-309

[2] Martin KR. Targeting apoptosis with dietary bioactive agents. Experimental Biology and Medicine. 2006;**231**:117-129

[3] James SJ, Muskhelishvili L, Gaylor DW, Turturro A, Hart R. Upregulation of apoptosis with dietary restriction: Implications for carcinogenesis. Environmental Health Perspectives. 1998;**106**(1):307-312

[4] Naik P, Karrim J, Hanahan D. The rise and fall of apoptosis during multistage tumorigenesis: Down-modulation contributes to tumour progression from angiogenic progenitors. Genes and Development. 1996;**10**:2105-2116

[5] Lijinsky W. Chemistry and Biology of N-nitroso Compounds. Cambridge University Press; 1992

[6] Siddoo-Atwal C. Heavy metal carcinogenesis: A possible mechanistic role for apoptosis. Vegetos. 2017;**30**(Special). DOI: 10.5958/2229-4473.2017.00046.5

[7] Siddoo-Atwal C. AT, apoptosis, and cancer: A viewpoint. Indian Journal of Ecology. 2009;**36**(2):103-110

[8] Sun S, Hail N, Lotan R. Apoptosis as a novel target for cancer chemoprevention. Journal of the National Cancer Institute. 2004;**96**:662-678

[9] Lokshin R, Zakeri Z. Apoptosis, autophagy, and more. International Journal of Biochemistry and Cell Biology. 2004;**36**:2405-2419

[10] Danial N, Korsmeyer S. Cell death: Critical control points. Cell. 2004;**116**:205-219

[11] Susin SS, Lorenzo HK, Zamzami N, Marzo I, Snow BE, Brothers GM, et al. Molecular characterization of mitochondrial apoptosis-inducing factor. Nature. 1999;**397**:441-446

[12] Siddoo-Atwal C, Atwal AS. A possible role for honey bee products in the detoxification of mycotoxins. ISHS Acta Horticulturae. 2012;**963**:237-245 (I International Symposium on Mycotoxins in Nuts and Dried Fruits)

[13] Siddoo-Atwal C. Chapter 8–Electromagnetic radiation from cellphone towers: A possible health hazard for birds, bees, and humans. In: Tutar Y, Tutar L, editors. Current Understanding of Apoptosis. INTECHOPEN; 2018

[14] Van Hogerlinden M, Rozell BL, Ahrlund-Richter L, ToftgArd R. Squamous cell carcinomas and increased apoptosis in skin with inhibited Rel/nuclear factor-κB signaling. Cancer Research. 1999;**59**:3299-3303

[15] Siddoo-Atwal C. A New Approach to Cancer Risk Assessment: An Overview. Lambert Academic Publishing (OmniScriptum); 2017

[16] Galanello R, Origa R. Beta-thalassemia. Orphanet Journal of Rare Diseases. 2010;**5**:11. DOI: 10.1186/1750-1172-5-11

[17] Cao A, Moi P. Regulation of the globin genes. Pediatric Research. 2002;**51**(4):415-421

[18] Nordermeer D, de Laat W. Joining the loops: Beta-globin gene regulation. IUBMB Life. 2008;**60**(12):824-833

[19] Ho PJ. The regulation of β globin gene expression and β thalassemia. Pathology. 1999;**31**:315-324

[20] Ikonomi P, Noguchi CT, Miller W, Kassahun H, Hardison R, Schechter AN. Levels of GATA-1/GATA-2 transcription factors modulate expression of embryonic and fetal hemoglobins. Gene. 2001;**261**(2):277-287

[21] Ropero P, Erquiaga S, Arrizabalaga B, Perez G, de la Iglesia S, Torrejon MJ, et al. Phenotype of mutations in the promoter region of the β-globin gene. Journal of Clinical Pathology. 2017;**70**(10):874-878

[22] Giglioni B, Comi P, Ronchi A, Mantovani R, Ottolenghi S. The same nuclear proteins bind the proximal CACCC box of the human beta-globin promoter and a similar sequence in the enhancer. Biochemical and Biophysical Research Communications. 1989;**164**(1):149-155

[23] Vetter B, Schwarz C, Kohne E, Kulozik AE. Beta-thalassaemia in the immigrant and non-immigrant German populations. British Journal of Haematology. 1997;**97**(2):266-272

[24] Kukreti R, B-Rao C, Das SK, De M, Talukder G, Vaz F, et al. Study of the single nucleotide polymorphism (SNP) at the palindromic dequence of hypersensitive site (HS)4 of the human b-globin locus control region (LCR) in Indian population. American Journal of Hematology. 2002;**69**:77-79

[25] Chandra RG. Indo-Greek Jewellery. New Delhi: Abhinav Publications; 1979

[26] Widemann F. Maues King of Taxila: An Indo-Greek Kingdom with a Saka King. East and West. 2003;**53**(1/4):95-125

[27] Bernard P. Chapter 4: The Greek Kingdoms of Central Asia. In: Harmatta J, editor. History of Civilizations of Central Asia. UNESCO Publishing; 1994. ISBN 978-92-3-102846-5

[28] Chintala S, Li W, Lamoreux ML, Ito S, Wakamatsu K, Sviderskaya EV, et al. Slc7a11 gene controls production of pheomelanin pigment and proliferation of cultured cells. Proceedings of the National Academy of Sciences of the United States of America. 2005;**102**(31):10964-10969

[29] Braun-Falco O, Plewig G, Wolff HH, Burgdorf WHC. Dermatology. 2nd ed. New York: Springer-Verlag Berlin Heidelberg; 1996

[30] Viprakasit V, Gibbons RJ, Broughton BC, Tolmie JL, Brown D, Lunt P, et al. Mutations in the general transcription factor TFIIH result in beta-thalassaemia in individuals with trichothiodystrophy. Human Molecular Genetics. 2001;**10**(24):2797-2802

[31] Lehmann AR, McGibbon D, Stefanini M. Xeroderma pigmentosum. Orphanet Journal of Rare Diseases. 2011;**6**:70. DOI: 10.1186/1750-1172-6-70

[32] Riou L, Eveno E, Van Hoffen A, Van Zeeland AA, Sarasin A, Mullenders LHF. Differential repair of the two major UV-induced photolesions in trichothiodystrophy fibroblasts. Cancer Research. 2004;**64**(3):889-894

[33] Lima-Bessa KM, Menck CFM. Skin cancer: Lights on genome lesions. Current Biology. 2005;**15**(Issue 2): R58-R61

[34] Nakajima S, Lan L, Kanno S-I, Takao M, Yamamoto K, Eker APM, et al. UV light-induced DNA damage and tolerance for the survival of nucleotide excision repair-deficient human cells. The Journal of Biological Chemistry. 2004;**279**:46674-46677

[35] Kraemer KH, Lee MM, Scotto JS. Xeroderma pigmentosum cutaneous, ocular, and neurologic abnormalities in 830 published cases. Archives of Dermatology. 1987;**123**(2):241-250

[36] Nelson HH, Kelsey KT, Mott LA, Karagas MR. The XRCC1 Arg399Gln polymorphism, sunburn, and non-melanoma cancer. Cancer Research. 2002;**62**:152-155

[37] Han J, Colditz GA, Samson LD, Hunter DJ. Polymorphisms in DNA double-strand break repair genes and skin cancer risk. Cancer Research. 2004;**64**:3009-3013

[38] Winsey SL, Haldar NA, Marsh HP, Bunce M, Marshall SE, Harris AL, et al. A variant within the DNA repair gene XRCC3 is associated with the development of melanoma skin cancer. Cancer Research. 2000;**60**:5612-5616

[39] Justenhoven C, Hamann V, Pesch B, Harth U, Rabstein S, Baisch C, et al. ERCC2 genotypes and a corresponding haplotype are linked with breast cancer risk in a German population. Cancer Epidemiology, Biomarkers and Prevention. 2004;**13**:2059-2064

[40] Smedby KE, Lindgren CM, Hjalgrim H, Humphreys K, Sholkopf C, Chang ET, et al. Variation in DNA repair genes *ERCC2, XRCC1*, and *XRCC3* and risk of follicular lymphoma. Cancer Epidemiology, Biomarkers and Prevention. 2006;**15**(2):258-265

[41] Voso M, Fabiani E, D'Alo F, Guidi F, Di Ruscio A, Sica S, et al. Increased risk of acute myeloid leukaemia due to polymorphisms in detoxification and DNA repair enzymes. Annals of Oncology. 2007;**18**(9):1523-1528

[42] Oetting WS, King RA. Molecular basis of albinism: Mutations and polymorphisms of pigmentation genes associated with albinism. Human Mutation. 1999;**13**(2):99-115

[43] Kromberg JGR, Castle D, Zwane EM, Jenkins T. Albinism and skin cancer in Southern Africa. Clinical Genetics. 1989;**36**:43-52

[44] De Gruijl FR, Forbes PD. UV-induced skin cancer in a hairless mouse model. BioEssays. 1995;**17**(7):651-661

[45] Taylor AM, Metcalfe JA, Thick J, Mak YF. Leukemia and lymphoma in Ataxia telangiectasia. Blood. 1996;**87**(2):423-438

[46] Takagi M, Delia D, Chessa L, Iwata S, Shigeta T, Kanke Y, et al. Defective control of apoptosis, radiosensitivity, and spindle checkpoint in ataxia telangiectasia. Cancer Research. 1998;**58**(21):4923-4929

[47] Savitsky K, Bar SA, Gilad S, Rotman G, Ziv Y, Vanagaite L, et al. A single ataxia telangiectasia gene with a product similar to PI-3 kinase. Science. 1995;**268**(5218):1749-1753

[48] Liao W-C, Haimovitz-Friedman A, Persaud RS, McLoughlin M, Ehleiter D, Zhang N, et al. Ataxia telangiectasia-mutated gene product inhibits DNA damage-induced apoptosis via ceramide synthase. Journal of Biological Chemistry. 1999;**274**(25):17908-17917

[49] Siddoo-Atwal C, Rosin MP, Haas AL. Elevation of interferon β-inducible proteins in Ataxia telangiectasia cells. Cancer Research. 1996;**56**:443-447

[50] Duchaud E, Ridet A, Stoppa-Lyonnet D, Janin N, Moustacchi E, Rosselli F. Deregulated apoptosis in Ataxia-telangiectasia: Association with clinical stigmata and radiosensitivity. Cancer Research. 1996;**56**:1400-1404

[51] Gao B. Cytokines, STATS and liver disease. Cellular & Molecular Immunology. 2005;**2**(2):92-100

[52] Jung M, Zhang Y, Lee S, Dritschilo A. Correction of radiation sensitivity in Ataxia telangiectasia cells by a

truncated I Kappa B-alpha. Science. 1995;**268**:1619-1621

[53] Rieux-Laucat F, Le Deist F, Fischer A. Autoimmune lymphoproliferative syndromes: Genetic defects of apoptosis pathways. Cell Death and Differentiation. 2003;**10**:124-133